Gluten-Free in Five Minutes

Also by Roben Ryberg:

The Ultimate Gluten-Free Cookie Book

You Won't Believe It's Gluten-Free!

The Gluten-Free Kitchen

Recipes by Roben Ryberg:

Eating for Autism

Gluten-Free in Five Minutes

123 Rapid Recipes for Breads, Rolls, Cakes, Muffins, and More

Roben Ryberg

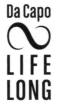

Da Capo

LIFE LONG

A Member of the Perseus Books Group

Design by Jill Shaffer
Set in 12-pt. Chaparral Light by Eclipse Publishing Services

Cataloging-in-Publication data for this book is available
from the Library of Congress.

First Da Capo Press edition 2011
ISBN: 978-0-7382-1462-7
Library of Congress Control Number: 2011927206

Published by Da Capo Press
A Member of the Perseus Books Group
www.dacapopress.com

Da Capo Press books are available at special discounts for bulk purchases in the U.S. by corporations, institutions, and other organizations. For more information, please contact the Special Markets Department at the Perseus Books Group, 2300 Chestnut Street, Suite 200, Philadelphia, PA, 19103, or call (800) 810-4145, ext. 5000, or e-mail special.markets@perseusbooks.com.

Note: This book is intended only as an informative guide for those wishing to know more about health issues. In no way is this book intended to replace, countermand, or conflict with the advice given to you by your own physician. The ultimate decision concerning care should be made between you and your doctor. We strongly recommend you follow his or her advice. Information in this book is general and is offered with no guarantees on the part of the authors or Da Capo Press. The authors and publisher disclaim all liability in connection with the use of this book.

10 9 8 7 6 5 4 3 2 1

Dedicated to everyone who believes in the impossible.
And thankful for God, friends, and family who
make it possible.

Contents

Photographs appear following page 74

Acknowledgments

I'd like to thank three of the youngest first testers of the chocolate cakes in this book, Braden, Corice, and Carter. Gluten-free or not, these kids know food!

Thank you to my other young friends, Ajaya, Tess, and Maddie, for grabbing the nearest stools in my kitchen to see what's cooking and give the latest recipes a try!

Thank you to my foodie friends, Cassandra, Stacie, and Sara. To my children for their amazing support. And to my dear friends, who accept my newest food science theories and are happy to share their taste buds and feedback.

And finally, to the people at Da Capo, especially Katie, who somehow take my words and recipes and turn them into a work of art worthy of a bookstore and your kitchen.

Foreword

As a dietitian and a person with celiac disease, I have often counseled patients new to gluten-free living with the news: "You'll have to learn to cook. Not because you want to, but because you have to . . . it is the only way to have the foods you want." Gluten-free, readymade products and mixes are more expensive than their wheat counterparts. Cooking gluten-free helps to control costs, allows you to create foods that you can eat if you have other food sensitivities, and provides fresh foods.

Of course, cooking from scratch isn't always practical. I remember a time when my daughter wanted an Easy Bake Oven for her birthday. Life was so busy, I thought, "Mommy wants an Easy Bake Oven, too." How I loved the microwave then and I still love it today. I learned to cook meats without turning them to rubber and to steam vegetables just right. However, what I couldn't do was prepare my favorite gluten-free foods—muffins, cupcakes, or even a casserole. For these items I either went without or resorted to a day of baking to have these foods on hand. This also meant having a pantry filled with specialty flours and gums, a separate set of pans and utensils, and time—lots of time!

Convenience has become a way of life. We want food fast, we want it now, and we don't always want to have to work to get it. Some people use their oven to store pots and pans they never use; others frequently order take-out. Those of us living gluten-free are no different. Few people have much time these days to do a lot of cooking. Because it's just plain easier to choose convenience over preparing meals, like other Americans, those of us who must live gluten-free don't have the healthiest diet when we live fast-paced lives—but the health consequences of resorting to take-out or fast food restaurants are even more serious.

Now, Roben Ryberg has changed all that. With *Gluten-Free in Five Minutes*, she has combined a few simple, common ingredients into amazingly easy gluten-free dishes, baked goods, and snacks you can make in the MICROWAVE! (My favorite is the cornbread, which is wonderfully moist.) Finally, I can have my cake made from scratch and eat it when I want it, too. This book provides the luxury of convenience with homemade goodness and healthier lower-cost foods. It is a must for anyone who needs to prepare quick and safe foods using little time and equipment.

The number of people living gluten-free has increased significantly in the last 10 years, largely due to increased awareness and medical and public education about celiac disease. The estimated prevalence of celiac disease—an autoimmune disorder that can lead to damage of the small intestine and malabsorption and malnutrition—in the United States is 1 in 100 people. In addition, a new set of conditions has emerged, known collectively as non-celiac gluten intolerances. The number of people with non-celiac gluten intolerances is estimated to be seven to eight times the 3 to 4 million people with celiac disease. (Non-celiac gluten intolerances are a general reaction to gluten but are not autoimmune, nor do these conditions damage the small intestine.) The outward symptoms for all gluten-sensitive conditions can be very similar to a number of other GI problems, making it hard to diagnose them.

No matter the cause, anyone requiring a gluten-free diet for medical reasons has no other treatment options. To stay healthy, they must follow a gluten-free diet for life.

Ryberg has found a way to address a real need. *Gluten-Free in Five Minutes* is a great resource for anyone who wants to follow a healthier gluten-free diet but has a very busy lifestyle; for anyone who wants to cook but needs meals to be quick to prepare; or for anyone who does not have the typical bevy of gluten-free flours and equipment on hand to bake from scratch. A handful of common ingredients, a microwave, and a few minutes—now that is all it takes to have delicious gluten-free food.

Cynthia Kupper, RD, Executive Director
Gluten Intolerance Group of North America

Introduction

There are moments in all of our lives when we feel compelled to reach for the impossible, think outside the box, and walk on the wild side. This is one of those moments.

Twenty years ago, when I first started creating gluten-free recipes, most gluten-free baked goods were not so tasty and were often heavy, gritty, or dry in texture. Since then, the industry-standard approach has been to use blends of three or more alternative grains to mimic wheat flour. As gluten-free baking evolved, the food became better—but the process became increasingly complicated and time-consuming for the home cook.

Now, with just a few ordinary ingredients, one gluten-free flour, a bowl, a fork, and a microwave, you can make delicious single-servings of breads, rolls, cakes, tortillas, and much more. Together we will make really tasty gluten-free food, astoundingly fast. Now you can quickly prepare that sandwich for lunch—including the bread—or have a piece of chocolate cake right when you crave it. *Gluten-Free in Five Minutes* will show you how.

People like great fresh food. I know I do. Unfortunately, special diets often mean settling for less—going without or purchasing packages of gluten-free breads, rolls, and cakes at great expense, hoping they'll be edible. Sounds appetizing already! I picture the scene in my head: *Where are those $2.00 (each) rolls? Oh yes, let me dig them out of the freezer, defrost them, and then toast them just a bit. Maybe this will help them taste better . . . or not.* Otherwise, we buy or mix pricey flour blends that take up lots of cabinet space, and we bake a whole loaf of bread knowing most of it will go into the freezer. If you are new to the gluten-free diet, it may seem like I am joking. If you already live the diet, you know it is reality.

Of course, I'm grateful that these days, one can go to the store and find better gluten-free product labeling and more foods available than ever before. But we pay dearly for the convenience.

Gluten-Free in Five Minutes gives you an amazing alternative. Now you can have two fabulous slices of fresh bread, truly ready in minutes. You can have dessert every night if you want it. These baked goods are moist, fresh, delicious, and no more freezer burn. But most importantly, these recipes give you social freedom. Maybe there's a dinner party you'd like to attend, but you need to bring something safe to eat. Your child receives a last-minute invitation for a party and he wants to have cake too, "like everyone else." A barbecue is happening down the street and it would be nice to grab a hot dog or hamburger roll. Or maybe you'd just like to be able to eat with friends without having to plan too far in advance. All that is possible!

About the Gluten-Free Diet

A gluten-free diet may be recommended for a variety of reasons: diagnosis of celiac disease (either by blood test or intestinal biopsy); dermatitis herpetiformis (DH), a skin manifestation of celiac disease; gluten intolerance; allergic reaction to ingestion of wheat; autism, Crohn's disease, or another autoimmune disease. Some people spend years searching for understanding of their medical issues. Weight loss, weight gain, diarrhea, malnutrition, gastro-intestinal symptoms, fatigue, headaches, and vitamin deficiencies are among the more common symptoms. Mild and atypical symptoms present as well.

Adhering to a gluten-free diet requires the strict avoidance of all wheat, rye, contaminated oats (cross-contaminated from field to factory), and barley. It is a simple prescription that can be very difficult to implement as wheat seems to be everywhere. It is obvious that some foods contain wheat (or rye, oats, barley), like breads, cakes, and cookies. But it is important to look closely in foods that you wouldn't suspect of having an offending ingredient. Check chips, soy sauce, soups, granola bars, sauces, spice blends, condiments, and many other foods! Federal regulations mandating that manufacturers disclose whether their products contain major food allergens (e.g., milk, eggs, fish, crustacean shellfish, tree nuts, wheat, peanuts, and soybeans) have recently made food ingredient labels easier to decipher for dietary concerns. It is hoped that the Food and Drug Administration will soon have a defined and imple-mented standard for "gluten-free" as well.

Simple, Safe, Fast, Good

With all my cookbooks, my goals have been simple: make it taste good, make it safe, and make it easy. That has never changed, and *Gluten-Free in Five Minutes* is no exception. However, my food science interpretation has evolved dramat-ically. Twenty years ago, had someone said I would be making light, delicious cake or bread using only brown rice flour or sorghum flour I wouldn't have believed them. Today it is reality. Incredible though it may seem, you really can use a microwave to make everyday baked goods!

One last note: While I do have several "non-baked" foods in here, this book is not a "how to make *everything* in the microwave" book. But what it does, it does extremely well—cakes, breads, cobblers, and more. It is the answer for quick servings of everyday foods you might be missing. In addition, recipes use just one flour, no xanthan gum or other binders are necessary, and many recipes are dairy-free as well. These whole grain breads and baked goods don't crumble and they taste great. With the Extreme Chocolate Cake recipe, you don't even need flour—just cocoa! And when the first strawberries of the season are at your market and you just can't resist, you can enjoy them with a Pound Cake, Chiffon Cake, or Angel Food Cake.

Whether you are a college student hoping to have safe food in your dorm, a mom who packs a child's lunch every day, a healthcare professional making food for a patient, a restaurateur wanting to meet the needs of a special customer, or simply a regular person hungry for one great serving of cake, welcome to the insanely fast side of eating well!

CHAPTER 1

Kitchen and Baking

Cooking Safely

For those who must avoid gluten, there are two primary areas of food concern. The first is ingredients, and the second is cross-contamination.

The recipes in this book call for very common ingredients and use only one gluten-free flour at a time—usually brown rice flour or sorghum flour. Unlike many other gluten-free recipes, for these you do not need the often-used specialty binder xanthan gum. This is especially nice for people who must avoid xanthan gum due to sensitivity (because it is often produced from a corn-sugar foundation).

The second area of food concern is cross-contamination. Simply put, your gluten-free ingredients and finished dishes should never come into contact with anything that has had contact with unsafe foods. Here's a helpful list for your kitchen.

1. Do you work on a clean surface? Be sure your countertops and cutting boards (and utensils and bowls) are freshly wiped or covered with a piece of foil. And that wiping cloth needs to be very clean too!

2. Are there crumbs in the silverware drawer? Crumbs of any kind must be avoided. It is not okay to simply brush them aside as even a minute amount of gluten can harm the intestine of someone with celiac disease. The cleaner your diet, the better you should feel.

3. Has that toaster/toaster oven been used for regular bread? If so, you either need a new, dedicated toaster, or toaster bags. (Please see the listing of gluten-free resources in the Appendix.)

4. Are your condiments yours alone? A knife touching regular toast then your butter makes your butter unsafe. Ditto for everything in your fridge.

5. Are your mixing and baking tools dedicated to your gluten-free cooking? If not, be sure they are meticulously clean!

6. Are your oven mitts, kitchen towels, and apron (if you use one) freshly washed? You don't want a wayward crumb or flour dust to contaminate your beautiful food!

Tools

Fortunately, few specialty tools are needed for gluten-free cooking in the microwave.

FOR MIXING:

One 2-cup capacity Pyrex or other similarly sized glass measuring cup
or mug

1 fork

1 knife (use backside to level ingredients in measuring spoons)

1 rubber spatula

1 set of any major name-brand measuring spoons (a set that includes a
⅛ teaspoon measure is especially nice)

FOR CHOPPING:

sharp knife

cutting board (not used with gluten-containing foods)

FOR MICROWAVING:

Microwave: All recipes were tested using a Whirlpool 1,000-watt microwave. There is a rhythm to the cooking times in this book. Most recipes
cook on high for 2 minutes. Please adjust cooking times based upon
the results using your microwave since each one is just a little different.
Incremental adjustments of no more than 15 seconds, more or less,
should be utilized as the basis for any cooking time changes.

Two 1-cup capacity Pyrex or other microwave-safe baking dishes (preferably
with straight sides)

One 2-cup capacity Pyrex or other microwave-safe baking dish (preferably
with straight sides)

One square 2-cup capacity Pyrex or other microwave-safe baking dish
(available online and in larger kitchen supply stores)

1 microwave-safe butter dish (inverted top used for making hot dog rolls)

1 microwave-safe plate

1 plain glass shot glass (to use in making bagels)

1 or 2 potholders

NICE EXTRAS TO HAVE ON HAND:

New toaster dedicated to gluten-free foods only or toaster bags

Pretty microwave-safe bowls for cooking and serving

Toaster oven for crisping pizza crust and bagels

Pan for making French Toast Circles (page 19) (only recipe requiring a pan)

Pantry Ingredients

Flours

Brown rice flour and sorghum flour are the primary flours used in this book. White rice flour has been used when lightness of texture and color are very important. Cornstarch and/or cornmeal have been used for variety.

Brown rice flour and white rice flour. Bob's Red Mill brand has been used exclusively in testing recipes in this book. This brand is available in most larger grocery stores and health food stores and is also available online. See the Appendix for ordering information.

Cornstarch and/or cornmeal. Please note that some brands are not produced in dedicated gluten-free facilities, which means there is some risk of cross-contamination. Calling the manufacturer (most list a phone number on the package) is the best way to evaluate any cross-contamination risk. Cornstarch and cornmeal are available in nearly all grocery stores.

Sorghum flour. Bob's Red Mill brand has been used exclusively in testing recipes in this book. This brand is available in most larger grocery stores and health food stores as well as online. Ordering information can be found in the Appendix.

Other Ingredients

Applesauce. Any brand should be fine. White House brand was used in testing all recipes in this book.

Baby food. Beech-Nut brand is preferred. I think it tastes better.

Baking powder. I used Rumford baking powder exclusively in creating and testing recipes in this book. It is manufactured by Clabber Girl and is available in most grocery stores and online; see the Appendix for ordering information. Please note that different brands of baking powder act differently! Some have more action in the bowl (like Rumford) while others have more action in the oven. Using a different brand could make a baked item fall or collapse. Should this happen, reduce the amount of baking powder by at least 25 percent.

Baking soda. Arm & Hammer is my favorite and is available in nearly all grocery stores.

Butter. Use any brand, lightly salted.

Cocoa powder. I recommend Hershey's for best flavor, available in nearly all grocery stores.

Cream cheese. Philadelphia is available in nearly all grocery stores.

Eggs. Use any brand, size large.

Milk. Recipes were created with 2% milk. Any brand can be used.

Nonstick cooking spray. I use the canola version of Pam, but any brand that is gluten-free should be fine.

Oatmeal. Be sure to use a brand of oats specifically labeled *gluten-free*. Cross-contamination is common among major national brands as mills and trucks are used for processing and transporting grains that are not gluten-free. Certified gluten-free oats are available through some grocery stores, health food stores, and online. See the Appendix for suppliers.

Oils. Canola oil and olive oil, any brand. Extra virgin olive oil has stronger flavor and is beneficial in the recipes suggesting its use.

Salad dressing. Use any brand that is gluten-free, but you must read ingredient listings to be sure that the dressing is truly gluten free. Wheat should be plainly listed if used as an ingredient.

Salt. Use any brand, but I find sea salt especially nice.

Spices, flavorings, and extracts. I recommend McCormick brand or any other brands that are gluten-free. See the Appendix for information on ordering butterscotch flavoring oil if you make the one snack cake using this flavoring.

Sour cream. Most brands; be sure to check ingredient label to be sure it is wheat-free. I do not like to use nonfat sour cream.

Sugar: white, brown, and confectioner's. All should be gluten-free, but double-check the labels!

Vinegar. Use apple cider vinegar, any brand. Be careful of flavored vinegars, however, as they may include hidden gluten.

Xanthan gum. This ingredient is *not* used in the recipes in this book!

Yogurt. Any brand plain, lowfat yogurt. I do not like to use nonfat yogurt in baking.

Microwave Baking Helpful Hints

Should you find yourself scratching your head wondering what went wrong with one of these simple recipes, I have a few insights that may be helpful.

1. *Baked item is too moist and seems undercooked.* Your cooking time needs to be extended. Try an additional 15 seconds. And if your microwave is really underpowered, try 15 seconds more after that.

2. *Baked item is a little dry.* Your cooking time needs to be decreased. Try using 15 seconds less. Your baked items should never be dry.

3. *Baked item collapses.* You may be using a different brand of baking powder than I did! If you are not using Rumford, decrease baking powder by 25 percent.

4. *Baked item overflows baking dish.* Your baking dish may be too small or you may be using a different brand of baking powder. First check the size of your baking dish. A slightly larger dish can make a big difference! Second, check your brand of baking powder. If it is not Rumford, decrease baking powder by 25 percent.

CHAPTER 2

Breakfast

Breakfast is a great way to start or end the day.

My favorite recipe in this chapter is Eggs Florentine. Sophisticated and delicious, make it, including the English Muffin (pages 16–18), when you want to pamper yourself or another special someone. In my opinion, a consistently perfect poached egg is impressive!

You may also wish to consider making Crepes (page 156) or Cinnamon Raisin Bread (pages 25–26) for breakfast as well.

And, as a final note, the Coffee Cake recipe (page 13) in this chapter will rival any you've ever eaten.

Bagel

(brown rice flour)
MAKES 1 BAGEL

✦

*Don't forget to use an inverted shot glass in the middle of your
Pyrex dish for the pretty bagel shape! This brown rice bagel is
a very mild bagel and is denser than the sorghum version.*

1 egg white

1 tablespoon canola oil

1½ tablespoons applesauce

1/16 teaspoon salt

2½ tablespoons brown rice
flour

¼ teaspoon baking powder

¼ teaspoon sugar

Baked in: 2-cup ramekin or other
straight-sided microwave-safe bowl with
a plain, microwave-safe shot glass inverted in the center of the baking dish

1. In small bowl or cup, briefly beat
   egg white until frothy (with varying
   bubble sizes).

2. Add remaining ingredients and mix
   well to combine.

3. Spray 2-cup ramekin with nonstick
   cooking spray. Spray microwave-safe
   shot glass with nonstick cooking
   spray. Place shot glass in center of
   ramekin.

4. Pour batter into ramekin and tap
   base to level batter.

5. Microwave on high for 2 minutes.
   Bagel will rise and then settle.

6. Gently remove from dish and cool.

7. Toast prior to serving for best crust.

Note: If you are toasting your bagel in a toaster oven, spray or sprinkle the
outside with lightly salted water for better exterior crust. These bagels are
better at room temperature than hot. Strange, but true.

Bagel

(sorghum flour)
MAKES 1 BAGEL

*This bagel must be toasted to get the crispy exterior, which isn't quite
like a real bagel. But the interior is dense with the tight crumb of a lighter
commercial-style bagel. Use an inverted shot glass in the middle
of your Pyrex bowl to create that bagel shape!*

1 egg white

1 tablespoon canola oil

1½ tablespoons applesauce

¹⁄₁₆ teaspoon salt

2 tablespoons sorghum flour

¼ teaspoon baking powder

¼ teaspoon sugar

Baked in: 2-cup ramekin or other straight-sided microwave-safe bowl, with a plain, microwave-safe shot glass in the center of the baking dish

1. In a small bowl or cup, briefly beat egg white until frothy (with varying bubble sizes).

2. Add remaining ingredients and mix well to combine.

3. Spray 2-cup ramekin with nonstick cooking spray. Spray microwave-safe shot glass with nonstick cooking spray. Place shot glass in center of ramekin.

4. Pour batter into ramekin and tap base to level batter.

5. Microwave on high for 2 minutes. Bagel will rise and then settle.

6. Gently remove from dish and cool.

7. Toast prior to serving for best crust.

Coffee Cake

(brown rice flour)
SERVES 2

In order to make a crispy cinnamon topping, a few gluten-free animal crackers are crushed and mixed with cinnamon and sugar. Feel free to substitute any crisp gluten-free cookie in their place. This is a bona fide, tasty coffee cake!

1 egg

1 tablespoon canola oil

3 tablespoons applesauce

1/16 teaspoon salt

3 tablespoons brown rice flour

1/2 teaspoon baking powder

1 tablespoon plus 1 teaspoon sugar

1/8 teaspoon vanilla

TOPPING:

10 gluten-free animal crackers, crushed or 2 1/2 tablespoons other crisp cookie crushed

1/4 teaspoon cinnamon

1 teaspoon brown sugar

Baked in: 2-cup ramekin or other straight-sided microwave-safe bowl

1. In a small bowl or cup, briefly beat egg until almost uniform in color.

2. Add remaining ingredients and mix well to combine.

3. Spray 2-cup ramekin with nonstick cooking spray.

4. Pour batter into ramekin and tap base to level batter. Set aside.

5. Combine topping ingredients.

6. Sprinkle over top of batter and swirl into batter with knife or spoon. Some topping should remain on the top.

7. Microwave on high for 2 minutes. Cake will rise and then settle a little during baking.

8. Gently remove from dish (keeping cake upright) and cool.

Eggs Benedict

SERVES 2

*By combining three recipes in this book, you can create
this classic gourmet breakfast dish!*

1 English Muffin, toasted and split (pages 16–18)

2 thick slices of pre-cooked ham

Hollandaise Sauce (page 73)

2 poached eggs (page 21)

1. Prepare English Muffin and toast it.

2. Place halves on two serving plates.

3. On separate plate, microwave ham slices for 30 seconds to warm. Place on top of English Muffin halves.

4. Prepare Hollandaise Sauce and set aside.

5. Prepare poached eggs and place on top of ham slices.

6. Pour Hollandaise Sauce over top.

Eggs Florentine

SERVES 1

There is a beautiful resort in Western Maryland called Rocky Gap. Overlooking the lake one morning, I enjoyed this dish for breakfast. Although not traditional, a little Hollandaise Sauce (page 73) is phenomenal drizzled over this dish!

1 medium mushroom, any kind you like

$\frac{1}{16}$ teaspoon garlic salt

$\frac{1}{2}$ tablespoon butter

1 cup fresh baby spinach (measured by pressing firmly into cup)

1 tomato slice

1 poached egg (page 21)

sprinkling of Parmesan cheese

sprinkling of salt and pepper

1. Wash mushroom and slice into microwave-safe cup. Add garlic salt and butter.

2. Microwave on high for 1 minute.

3. Spread onto serving plate.

4. Wash spinach and place in microwave-safe cup. Spinach should be damp.

5. Microwave on high for 45 seconds.

6. Drain excess water. Pile spinach on top of mushrooms.

7. Place tomato slice on top of spinach.

8. Poach egg and place on top of tomato.

9. Sprinkle Parmesan cheese, salt, and pepper on top. Serve immediately.

Note: A plain white button mushroom would be a great introduction to someone new to eating mushrooms. A crimini mushroom would have more flavor. And a shiitake mushroom would be perfect for a mushroom enthusiast.

English Muffin

(brown rice flour)
MAKES 1 MUFFIN

This is a very neutral-tasting English muffin . . . a lot like ordinary English muffins. Toast it extra long for that crunchy exterior that is so delicious!

1 egg white

2 teaspoons canola oil

2 tablespoons applesauce

small pinch of salt

3 tablespoons brown rice flour

¼ teaspoon baking powder

⅛ teaspoon baking soda

½ teaspoon sugar

Baked in: 1-cup ramekin or other straight-sided microwave-safe bowl

1. In small bowl or cup, briefly beat egg white to frothy (bubbles of varying size).
2. Add remaining ingredients and mix well to combine.
3. Spray ramekin with nonstick cooking spray.
4. Pour batter into ramekin and tap base to level batter.
5. Microwave on high for 1 minute.
6. Gently remove from dish and allow to cool.
7. Split in half and toast before serving.

English Muffin

(cornmeal)
MAKES 1 MUFFIN

This English muffin is fairly light in texture with a definite, but pleasant, corn undertone. The nooks and crannies are formed from the froth of the beaten egg white!

1 egg white

2 teaspoons canola oil

2 tablespoons applesauce

small pinch of salt

3 tablespoons cornmeal

¼ teaspoon baking powder

⅛ teaspoon baking soda

¼ teaspoon sugar

Baked in: 1-cup ramekin or other straight-sided microwave-safe bowl

1. In small bowl or cup, briefly beat egg white to frothy (bubbles of varying size).

2. Add remaining ingredients and mix well to combine.

3. Spray ramekin with nonstick cooking spray.

4. Pour batter into ramekin and tap base to level batter.

5. Microwave on high for 1 minute.

6. Gently remove from dish and allow to cool.

7. Split in half and toast before serving.

English Muffin

(sorghum flour)
MAKES 1 MUFFIN

*If you like whole-grain flavor and a heavier, tighter crumb,
this English muffin may be your favorite!*

1 egg white

1 teaspoon canola oil

1½ tablespoons applesauce

¹⁄₁₆ teaspoon salt

4 tablespoons sorghum flour

¹⁄₁₆ teaspoon baking soda

Baked in: 1-cup ramekin or other straight-sided microwave-safe bowl

1. In small bowl or cup, briefly beat egg white to frothy (bubbles of varying size).

2. Add remaining ingredients and mix well to combine.

3. Spray ramekin with nonstick cooking spray.

4. Pour batter into ramekin and tap base to level batter.

5. Microwave on high for 1 minute.

6. Gently remove from dish and allow to cool.

7. Split in half and toast before serving.

French Toast Circles

*This recipe was tested using the Applesauce Bread (brown rice flour)
recipe on page 139, but almost any quick bread recipe in this book
would be delicious. Be ready for a wonderful breakfast.
Leftover slices are delicious warmed in a toaster.*

1 recipe Applesauce Bread
(brown rice flour) page 139,
prepared and cooled

2 eggs

¼ cup milk

several drops vanilla extract

1. Preheat griddle to 350°F or heat
   frying pan over medium heat.

2. Lightly coat griddle or pan with
   nonstick cooking spray (away from
   flame if using gas stove).

3. Slice Applesauce Bread horizontally
   into 3 round discs. Set aside.

4. Combine eggs, milk, and vanilla
   extract in shallow bowl and mix well.

5. Dip bread slices into egg mixture
   and coat well on both sides. You may
   have a little excess egg mixture.

6. Place slices onto heated griddle
   or pan. Cook for approximately
   2 minutes on each side, until lightly
   browned and cooked through.

7. Serve with syrup or jam as desired.

Breakfast

Pancake

(brown rice flour)
MAKES 1 PANCAKE

This soft and slightly sweet pancake isn't as flat and uniform in shape as a traditional pancake, but it sure is fast and tasty.

1 egg

1 tablespoon canola oil

1 tablespoon applesauce

1/16 teaspoon salt

2 1/2 tablespoons brown rice flour

1/2 teaspoon baking powder

1 teaspoon sugar

Baked on: microwave-safe dinner plate

1. In small bowl or cup, briefly beat egg until nearly uniform in color.

2. Add remaining ingredients and mix well to combine.

3. Spray microwave-safe plate with nonstick cooking spray.

4. Pour batter onto plate and spread into 5-inch circle. The pancake will spread during cooking.

6. Microwave on high for 2 minutes.

7. Remove from oven and flip over to allow bottom to dry a little.

8. Serve with syrup as desired.

Poached Egg

SERVES 1

Poached eggs are so delicious and easy to make in the microwave, yet I've never known anyone to make them this way. Use extreme care in making poached eggs in the microwave as eggs may "pop" if overcooked, and this danger increases dramatically if more than one egg is poached at a time!

1 cup water

1 egg

1. In 2-cup microwave-safe bowl or cup, microwave water on high for 1½ minutes, or until boiling.

2. Crack egg into boiling water and microwave on high for 1 minute. If you prefer egg firmer in texture, microwave on high for an additional 10 to 15 seconds.

3. Carefully remove poached egg and discard any frothy bits.

Note: In traditionally poached eggs, a little vinegar is often added to the water before poaching. I have tested making poached eggs in the microwave both with and without the vinegar with no noticeable difference.

CHAPTER 3

Breads

Every bread in this chapter is delicious. I had non-testers "testing" recipe after recipe, seeking to eat more of this bread or that bread. These breads can be made incredibly quickly—and they are just plain good!

Figuring out how to make fabulous (yes, I said *fabulous*!) breads and rolls in the microwave was difficult at first. It comes down to food science.

For those of you who are already bakers, you know that egg whites are drying. Egg yolks add richness. And, while I'm not forgetting that oil adds softness and applesauce adds structure (and

Note: When I'm being exceptionally picky and want slices of bread to look exactly like two slices from the middle of a loaf of bread, I simply cut off a very thin slice from each end and split the middle into two beautiful slices of bread.

moisture), the most important factor in gluten-free/microwave context is the egg yolk. Using only egg whites (as in my full-size bread recipes) does not give the structure or texture or even the appropriate "dryness" needed in these recipes. But, when I decided to stop thinking and go with my gut instinct to use the entire egg, formulations began to fall into place. Gluten-free food science has evolved dramatically over the last twenty years, yet we are just scratching the surface of using whole grains well. And treating foods differently when they are microwaved is a perfect example of this!

Probably the most difficult part of making these bread recipes is locating a microwave-safe square dish. After much searching, I found a heavy glass storage container by Glasslock with a "locking" lid. Its base is just a bit smaller than a traditional slice of bread and works perfectly for these recipes. I have located these containers in a number of kitchen supply stores and at amazon.com. You can use a round 2-cup Pyrex dish, but the square slices are really nice.

Cinnamon Raisin Bread

(brown rice flour)
MAKES 2 SLICES

This recipe makes wonderful cinnamon raisin bread.
Enjoy it toasted and topped with cream cheese.

1 egg

1 tablespoon canola oil

1½ tablespoons applesauce

1/16 teaspoon salt

2½ tablespoons brown rice
flour

½ teaspoon baking powder

½ teaspoon sugar

1 tablespoon raisins, minced

¼ teaspoon cinnamon

Baked in: 2-cup square ramekin or other straight-sided microwave-safe bowl

1. In small bowl or cup, briefly beat egg until nearly uniform in color.

2. Add remaining ingredients and mix well to combine.

3. Spray 2-cup ramekin with nonstick cooking spray.

4. Pour batter into ramekin and tap base to level batter.

5. Microwave on high for 2 minutes. Bread will rise and then settle.

6. Gently remove from dish and cool.

7. Slice in half horizontally.

Cinnamon Raisin Bread

(sorghum flour)
MAKES 2 SLICES

This bread has an understated cinnamon and raisin flavor.
Our taster didn't want to share and ate both slices!

1 egg

1 tablespoon canola oil

1½ tablespoons applesauce

¹⁄₁₆ teaspoon salt

2 tablespoons sorghum flour

½ teaspoon baking powder

½ teaspoon sugar

¼ teaspoon cinnamon

1 tablespoon raisins, minced

Baked in: 2-cup square ramekin or other straight-sided microwave-safe bowl

1. In small bowl or cup, briefly beat egg until nearly uniform in color.
2. Add remaining ingredients and mix well to combine.
3. Spray 2-cup ramekin with nonstick cooking spray.
4. Pour batter into ramekin and tap base to level batter.
5. Microwave on high for 2 minutes. Bread will rise and then settle.
6. Gently remove from dish and cool.
7. Slice in half horizontally.

Cornbread

(brown rice flour)
SERVES 2

For those of you who do not tolerate corn, this brown rice version is great with chili, chicken, or whatever! The texture is tight and slightly softer than corn-based cornbread. I like this version every bit as much as the classic.

1 egg

2 teaspoons canola oil

2 tablespoons applesauce

rounded 1/16 teaspoon salt

3 tablespoons brown rice flour

1/4 teaspoon baking powder

1/2 teaspoon sugar

Baked in: 2-cup ramekin or other straight-sided microwave-safe bowl

1. In small bowl or cup, briefly beat egg until almost uniform in color.

2. Add remaining ingredients and mix well to combine.

3. Spray 2-cup ramekin with nonstick cooking spray.

4. Pour batter into ramekin and tap base to level batter.

5. Microwave on high for 2 minutes. Bread will rise and then settle a little during baking.

6. Gently remove from dish, if desired, and cool.

Cornbread

(cornmeal)
SERVES 2

*This is a plain old cornbread recipe. If you prefer
a sweeter cornbread, increase the sugar just a little.*

1 egg

2 teaspoons canola oil

2 tablespoons applesauce

rounded $\frac{1}{16}$ teaspoon salt

3$\frac{1}{2}$ tablespoons cornmeal

$\frac{1}{4}$ teaspoon baking powder

$\frac{3}{4}$ teaspoon sugar

Baked in: 2-cup ramekin or other
straight-sided microwave-safe bowl

1. In small bowl or cup, briefly beat egg
   until almost uniform in color.
2. Add remaining ingredients and mix
   well to combine.
3. Spray 2-cup ramekin with nonstick
   cooking spray.
4. Pour batter into ramekin and tap
   base to level batter.
5. Microwave on high for 2 minutes.
   Bread will rise and then settle a little
   during baking.
6. Gently remove from dish, if desired,
   and cool.

28

Honey Oat Bread

(brown rice flour)
MAKES 2 SLICES

*This bread is sweet and mild in flavor. Although delicious as is,
it is especially nice toasted. The oats are cooked for just 15 seconds
before combining with the other ingredients to soften.
Please remember to buy a gluten-free brand of oats!*

1 tablespoon gluten-free oats

1 tablespoon water

1 egg

1 tablespoon canola oil

1 tablespoon applesauce

$\frac{1}{16}$ teaspoon salt

2$\frac{1}{2}$ tablespoons brown rice flour

$\frac{1}{2}$ teaspoon baking powder

1 tablespoon honey

Baked in: 2-cup square ramekin or other straight-sided microwave-safe bowl

1. In small microwave-safe bowl, combine oats and water. Stir.

2. Microwave on high for 15 seconds. Set aside.

3. In a small bowl or cup, briefly beat egg until nearly uniform in color.

4. Add remaining ingredients including oats mixture and mix well to combine.

5. Spray 2-cup ramekin with nonstick cooking spray.

6. Pour batter into ramekin and tap base to level batter.

7. Microwave on high for 2 minutes. Bread will rise and then settle.

8. Gently remove from dish and cool.

9. Slice in half horizontally.

Honey Oat Bread

(sorghum flour)
MAKES 2 SLICES

Honey and oats are the perfect way to soften the whole-grain taste of sorghum flour. Enjoy this bread as a roll or sliced!

1 tablespoon gluten-free oats

1 tablespoon water

1 egg

1 tablespoon canola oil

1 tablespoon applesauce

1/16 teaspoon salt

2 tablespoons sorghum flour

1/2 teaspoon baking powder

1 tablespoon honey

Baked in: 2-cup square ramekin or other straight-sided microwave-safe bowl

1. In small microwave-safe bowl, combine oats and water. Stir.

2. Microwave on high for 15 seconds. Set aside.

3. In small bowl or cup, briefly beat egg until nearly uniform in color.

4. Add remaining ingredients including oat mixture and mix well to combine.

5. Spray 2-cup ramekin with nonstick cooking spray.

6. Pour batter into ramekin and tap base to level batter.

7. Microwave on high for 2 minutes. Bread will rise and then settle.

8. Gently remove from dish and cool.

9. Slice in half horizontally, if desired.

Sandwich Bread

(brown rice flour)
MAKES 2 SLICES

✳

Great soft sandwich bread texture, and a mild taste, too!

1 egg

1 tablespoon canola oil

1½ tablespoons applesauce

1/16 teaspoon salt

2½ tablespoons brown rice flour

½ teaspoon baking powder

¼ teaspoon sugar

Baked in: 2-cup square ramekin or other straight-sided microwave-safe bowl

1. In small bowl or cup, briefly beat egg until nearly uniform in color.
2. Add remaining ingredients and mix well to combine.
3. Spray 2-cup ramekin with nonstick cooking spray.
4. Pour batter into ramekin and tap base to level batter.
5. Microwave on high for 2 minutes. Bread will rise and then settle.
6. Gently remove from dish and cool.
7. Slice in half horizontally.

Sandwich Bread

(cornstarch and cornmeal)
MAKES 2 SLICES

This is a relatively moist, tight-crumb bread that is mild and soft.

1 egg

1 tablespoon canola oil

1½ tablespoons applesauce

1/16 teaspoon salt

1 tablespoon cornstarch

1 tablespoon cornmeal

½ teaspoon baking powder

¾ teaspoon sugar

Baked in: 2-cup square ramekin or other straight-sided microwave-safe bowl

1. In small bowl or cup, briefly beat egg until nearly uniform in color.
2. Add remaining ingredients and mix well to combine.
3. Spray 2-cup ramekin with nonstick cooking spray.
4. Pour batter into ramekin and tap base to level batter.
5. Microwave on high for 2 minutes. Bread will rise and then settle.
6. Gently remove from dish and cool.
7. Slice in half horizontally.

Sandwich Bread

(sorghum flour)
MAKES 2 SLICES

This sandwich bread has a mild whole-grain taste and a tight crumb.

1 egg

1 tablespoon canola oil

1½ tablespoons applesauce

⅟₁₆ teaspoon salt

2 tablespoons sorghum flour

½ teaspoon baking powder

¼ teaspoon sugar

Baked in: 2-cup square ramekin or other straight-sided microwave-safe bowl

1. In small bowl or cup, briefly beat egg until nearly uniform in color.
2. Add remaining ingredients and mix well to combine.
3. Spray 2-cup ramekin with nonstick cooking spray.
4. Pour batter into ramekin and tap base to level batter.
5. Microwave on high for 2 minutes. Bread will rise and then settle.
6. Gently remove from dish and cool.
7. Slice in half horizontally.

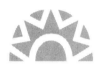

CHAPTER 4

Rolls

Like the breads in this book, these rolls are fabulous. Try one, try them all! Most of these rolls are moist and soft. The hamburger rolls are a little less moist, just as they should be. If you would like a crisp crust on any of these rolls, pop them in a toaster oven (or traditional oven) for a few minutes.

Best of all, you can be confident in making a sandwich for your lunch! These gluten-free rolls stay perfect and do not crumble.

Hamburger Roll

(brown rice flour)
MAKES 1 ROLL

A mild-tasting hamburger roll. I'd love to be more descriptive,
but it is just what you're looking to put a burger on.

1 egg

½ tablespoon canola oil

1 tablespoon applesauce

¹⁄₁₆ teaspoon salt

2 tablespoons brown rice flour

½ teaspoon baking powder

½ teaspoon sugar

Baked in: 2-cup ramekin or other straight-sided microwave-safe bowl

1. In small bowl or cup, briefly beat egg until almost uniform in color.

2. Add remaining ingredients and mix well to combine.

3. Spray 2-cup ramekin with nonstick cooking spray.

4. Pour batter into ramekin and tap base to level batter.

5. Microwave on high for 2 minutes. Roll will rise and then settle.

6. Gently remove from dish and cool.

Hamburger Roll

(cornstarch and cornmeal)
MAKES 1 ROLL

This is a straightforward hamburger roll. The taste and texture are pretty amazing. If you're wondering which roll to make for a burger, make this one!

1 egg

½ tablespoon canola oil

1 tablespoon applesauce

¹⁄₁₆ teaspoon salt

1 tablespoon cornstarch

1 tablespoon cornmeal

½ teaspoon baking powder

½ teaspoon sugar

Baked in: 2-cup ramekin or other straight-sided microwave-safe bowl

1. In small bowl or cup, briefly beat egg until almost uniform in color.

2. Add remaining ingredients and mix well to combine.

3. Spray 2-cup ramekin with nonstick cooking spray.

4. Pour batter into ramekin and tap base to level batter.

5. Microwave on high for 2 minutes. Roll will rise and then settle.

6. Gently remove from dish and cool.

Hamburger Roll

(sorghum flour)
MAKES 1 ROLL

This is a tasty whole-grain roll that is not too heavy and not too sweet.

1 egg

½ tablespoon canola oil

1 tablespoon applesauce

¹⁄₁₆ teaspoon salt

2 tablespoons sorghum flour

½ teaspoon baking powder

¼ teaspoon sugar

Baked in: 2-cup ramekin or other straight-sided microwave-safe bowl

1. In small bowl or cup, briefly beat egg until almost uniform in color.

2. Add remaining ingredients and mix well to combine.

3. Spray 2-cup ramekin with nonstick cooking spray.

4. Pour batter into ramekin and tap base to level batter.

5. Microwave on high for 2 minutes. Roll will rise and then settle.

6. Gently remove from dish and cool.

Hamburger Roll

(white rice flour)
MAKES 1 ROLL

The lightest in color and sweetest of the hamburger rolls.
Your gluten-eating friends are sure to like it as well.

1 egg

½ tablespoon canola oil

1 tablespoon applesauce

1/16 teaspoon salt

1 tablespoon plus 2 teaspoons white rice flour

½ teaspoon baking powder

¾ teaspoon sugar

Baked in: 2-cup ramekin or other straight-sided microwave-safe bowl

1. In small bowl or cup, briefly beat egg until almost uniform in color.

2. Add remaining ingredients and mix well to combine.

3. Spray 2-cup ramekin with nonstick cooking spray.

4. Pour batter into ramekin and tap base to level batter.

5. Microwave on high for 2 minutes. Roll will rise and then settle.

6. Gently remove from dish and cool.

Hot Dog Roll

(brown rice flour)
MAKES 1 ROLL

Ever want to join that barbecue down the street, but need a roll for that perfectly grilled hot dog? Not a problem anymore! This roll is made in the top half of a microwave-safe butter dish turned upside down. It is soft, slightly moister, and slightly denser than the hamburger rolls in this book.

1 egg

2 teaspoons canola oil

1 tablespoon applesauce

1/16 teaspoon salt

2 tablespoons brown rice flour

1/4 teaspoon baking powder

1/2 teaspoon sugar

Baked in: microwave-safe butter dish, upside-down

1. In small bowl or cup, briefly beat egg until almost uniform in color.

2. Add remaining ingredients and mix well to combine.

3. Spray top of microwave-safe butter dish with nonstick cooking spray.

4. Pour batter into dish and tap base to level batter.

5. Microwave on high for 1½ minutes. Roll will rise and then settle.

6. Gently remove from dish and cool.

Hot Dog Roll

(cornstarch and cornmeal)
MAKES 1 ROLL

This is a perfect hot dog roll—mild and tasting much like a traditional hot dog roll.

1 egg

2 teaspoons canola oil

1 tablespoon applesauce

$\frac{1}{16}$ teaspoon salt

1 tablespoon cornstarch

1 tablespoon cornmeal

scant $\frac{1}{4}$ teaspoon baking powder

$\frac{1}{2}$ teaspoon sugar

Baked in: microwave-safe butter dish, upside-down

1. In small bowl or cup, briefly beat egg until almost uniform in color.
2. Add remaining ingredients and mix well to combine.
3. Spray top of microwave-safe butter dish with nonstick cooking spray.
4. Pour batter into dish and tap base to level batter.
5. Microwave on high for 1½ minutes. Roll will rise and then settle.
6. Gently remove from dish and cool.

Hot Dog Roll

(sorghum flour)
MAKES 1 ROLL

*Like the other hot dog rolls in this book, this roll is made
in the top half of a microwave-safe butter dish turned upside down.
This is a lighter-textured hot dog roll.*

1 egg

2 teaspoons canola oil

1 tablespoon applesauce

1/16 teaspoon salt

2 tablespoons sorghum flour

scant 1/4 teaspoon baking
powder

1/4 teaspoon sugar

Baked in: microwave-safe butter dish,
upside-down

1. In small bowl or cup, briefly beat egg
   until almost uniform in color.

2. Add remaining ingredients and mix
   well to combine.

3. Spray top of microwave-safe butter
   dish with nonstick cooking spray.

4. Pour batter into dish and tap base to
   level batter.

5. Microwave on high for 1½ minutes.
   Roll will rise and then settle.

6. Gently remove from dish and cool.

Rolls

Italian Roll

(brown rice flour)
MAKES 1 ROLL

*Olive oil, garlic salt, and oregano are paired
to give this roll a nice Italian flavor.*

1 egg

1 tablespoon olive oil

1½ tablespoons applesauce

⅛ teaspoon garlic salt

2½ tablespoons brown rice flour

½ teaspoon baking powder

¼ teaspoon sugar

¼ teaspoon oregano or Italian seasoning

Baked in: 2-cup ramekin or other straight-sided microwave-safe bowl

1. In small bowl or cup, briefly beat egg until nearly uniform in color.

2. Add remaining ingredients and mix well to combine.

3. Spray 2-cup ramekin with nonstick cooking spray.

4. Pour batter into ramekin and tap base to level batter.

5. Microwave on high for 2 minutes. Roll will rise and then settle.

6. Gently remove from dish and cool.

Italian Roll

Like the brown rice version of the Italian Roll,
olive oil and oregano are used to flavor this roll.

1 egg

1 tablespoon olive oil

1½ tablespoons applesauce

⅛ teaspoon garlic salt

2 tablespoons sorghum flour

½ teaspoon baking powder

¼ teaspoon sugar

¼ teaspoon oregano or Italian seasoning

Baked in: 2-cup ramekin or other straight-sided microwave-safe bowl

1. In small bowl or cup, briefly beat egg until nearly uniform in color.
2. Add remaining ingredients and mix well to combine.
3. Spray 2-cup ramekin with nonstick cooking spray.
4. Pour batter into ramekin and tap base to level batter.
5. Microwave on high for 2 minutes. Roll will rise and then settle.
6. Gently remove from dish and cool.

Rolls

Onion Roll

(brown rice flour)
MAKES 1 ROLL

*This roll is soft and heavier in texture than
other rolls in this book. It is full of onion flavor!*

1 egg

1 tablespoon canola oil

1 tablespoon applesauce

$\frac{1}{16}$ teaspoon salt

2$\frac{1}{2}$ tablespoons brown rice
    flour

$\frac{1}{4}$ teaspoon baking powder

$\frac{1}{4}$ teaspoon sugar

1$\frac{1}{2}$ tablespoons minced onion

Baked in: 2-cup ramekin or other
straight-sided microwave-safe bowl

1. In small bowl or cup, briefly beat egg
until nearly uniform in color.

2. Add remaining ingredients and mix
well to combine.

3. Spray 2-cup ramekin with nonstick
cooking spray.

4. Pour batter into ramekin and tap
base to level batter.

5. Microwave on high for 2 minutes.
Roll will rise and then settle.

6. Gently remove from dish and cool.

Onion Roll

(sorghum flour)
MAKES 1 ROLL

*This roll would be delicious with
a grilled burger or other hearty fillings!*

1 egg

1 tablespoon canola oil

1 tablespoon applesauce

$\frac{1}{16}$ teaspoon salt

2 tablespoons sorghum flour

$\frac{1}{4}$ teaspoon baking powder

$\frac{1}{4}$ teaspoon sugar

$1\frac{1}{2}$ tablespoons minced onion

Baked in: 2-cup ramekin or other straight-sided microwave-safe bowl

1. In small bowl or cup, briefly beat egg until nearly uniform in color.

2. Add remaining ingredients and mix well to combine.

3. Spray 2-cup ramekin with nonstick cooking spray.

4. Pour batter into ramekin and tap base to level batter.

5. Microwave on high for 2 minutes. Roll will rise and then settle.

6. Gently remove from dish and cool.

Potato-style Roll

(brown rice flour)
MAKES 1 ROLL

This is the lightest-textured and most moist of the potato-style rolls. The flavor is slightly sweet and mild.

1 egg

1 tablespoon canola oil

2 tablespoons applesauce

$\frac{1}{16}$ teaspoon salt

2 tablespoons brown rice flour

$\frac{1}{2}$ teaspoon baking powder

1 teaspoon sugar

Baked in: 2-cup ramekin or other straight-sided microwave-safe bowl

1. In small bowl or cup, briefly beat egg until nearly uniform in color.

2. Add remaining ingredients and mix well to combine.

3. Spray 2-cup ramekin with nonstick cooking spray.

4. Pour batter into ramekin and tap base to level batter.

5. Microwave on high for 2 minutes. Roll will rise and then settle.

6. Gently remove from dish and cool.

Potato-style Roll

(white rice flour)
MAKES 1 ROLL

This roll is moister and more tender than a hamburger bun.
Bake this recipe in two 1-cup ramekins if you'd prefer dinner-size rolls.

1 egg

1 tablespoon canola oil

1 tablespoon applesauce

1/16 teaspoon salt

1 tablespoon plus 2 teaspoons
  white rice flour

1/2 teaspoon baking powder

1 teaspoon sugar

Baked in: 2-cup ramekin or two 1-cup ramekins for smaller rolls

1. In small bowl or cup, briefly beat egg until nearly uniform in color.

2. Add remaining ingredients and mix well to combine.

3. Spray 2-cup ramekin with nonstick cooking spray.

4. Pour batter into ramekin and tap base to level batter.

5. Microwave on high for 2 minutes. Roll will rise and then settle.

6. Gently remove from dish and cool.

Roll

(cornstarch and cornmeal)
MAKES 1 ROLL

This roll is very pleasant. It combines the flavor of cornbread with the texture of a roll. Be sure to use a ramekin that holds at least 1 cup to avoid overflow during baking.

1 egg white

½ tablespoon canola oil

2 tablespoons applesauce

¹⁄₁₆ teaspoon salt

1 tablespoon cornstarch

1 tablespoon cornmeal

½ teaspoon baking powder

Baked in: 1-cup ramekin or other straight-sided microwave-safe bowl. A slightly larger base makes for a nice burger-sized bun!

1. In small bowl or cup, briefly beat egg white until frothy (with varying bubble sizes).

2. Add remaining ingredients and mix well to combine.

3. Spray 1-cup ramekin with nonstick cooking spray.

4. Pour batter into ramekin and tap base to level batter.

5. Microwave on high for 2 minutes. Roll will rise and then settle.

6. Gently remove from dish and cool.

Roll

(sorghum flour)
MAKES 1 ROLL

The flavor of this roll is somewhere between that of whole wheat and corn, which is precisely the flavor of sorghum in breads! The roll is springy in texture.

1 egg white

1 tablespoon canola oil

2 tablespoons applesauce

¹⁄₁₆ teaspoon salt

3 tablespoons sorghum flour

½ teaspoon baking powder

¹⁄₃₂ teaspoon baking soda (little pinch)

TOPPING (OPTIONAL):

pinch of flaxseed meal

Baked in: 1-cup ramekin or other straight-sided microwave-safe bowl. A slightly larger base makes for a nice burger-sized bun!

1. In small bowl or cup, briefly beat egg white until frothy (with varying bubble sizes).

2. Add remaining ingredients and mix well to combine.

3. Spray 1-cup ramekin with nonstick cooking spray.

4. Pour batter into ramekin and tap base to level batter.

5. Microwave on high for 2 minutes. Roll will rise and then settle a little during baking.

6. Gently remove from dish and cool.

Sourdough Roll

(brown rice flour)
MAKES 1 ROLL

As the name suggests, this roll has a mild sourdough taste.

1 egg

1 tablespoon canola oil

1 tablespoon applesauce

1 teaspoon apple cider vinegar

1/16 teaspoon salt

2½ tablespoons brown rice flour

½ teaspoon baking powder

¼ teaspoon sugar

Baked in: 2-cup ramekin or other straight-sided microwave-safe bowl

1. In small bowl or cup, briefly beat egg until frothy (with varying bubble sizes).

2. Add remaining ingredients and mix well to combine.

3. Spray 2-cup ramekin with nonstick cooking spray.

4. Pour batter into ramekin and tap base to level batter.

5. Microwave on high for 2 minutes. Roll will rise and then settle.

6. Gently remove from dish and cool.

Sourdough Roll

(sorghum flour)
MAKES 1 ROLL

The vinegar in this recipe provides the sour taste, so no fermented yeast is required. For more sour taste, increase the vinegar to 1½ teaspoons.

1 egg

1 tablespoon canola oil

1 tablespoon applesauce

1 teaspoon apple cider vinegar

1/16 teaspoon salt

2 tablespoons sorghum flour

1/2 teaspoon baking powder

1/4 teaspoon sugar

Baked in: 2-cup ramekin or other straight-sided microwave-safe bowl

1. In small bowl or cup, briefly beat egg until frothy (with varying bubble sizes).

2. Add remaining ingredients and mix well to combine.

3. Spray 2-cup ramekin with nonstick cooking spray.

4. Pour batter into ramekin and tap base to level batter.

5. Microwave on high for 2 minutes. Roll will rise and then settle.

6. Gently remove from dish and cool.

CHAPTER 5

Flatbreads, Tortillas, and Pizza Crusts

As with breads and rolls, initially I was pretty nervous about being able to recreate appropriate textures for quick gluten-free flatbreads, tortillas, and pizza crusts. Would it be possible? But through subtle manipulation of very basic ingredients, we are able to do just that.

This is especially apparent in making flour tortillas. Unlike many other "bread" recipes, these tortilla recipes contain no applesauce for texture or oil to soften the texture of the grain. By omitting these ingredients, the texture of a flour tortilla is achieved, and the flavors of the flours come through clear and true.

Flatbread

(brown rice flour)
MAKES 1 FLATBREAD

Soft, squishy, and flat—just as a flatbread should be.
The flavor is very neutral and pleasant.

1 egg

1 tablespoon canola oil

1 tablespoon applesauce

$\frac{1}{16}$ teaspoon salt

2 tablespoons brown rice flour

$\frac{1}{2}$ teaspoon baking powder

$\frac{1}{8}$ teaspoon sugar

Baked on: microwave-safe dinner plate

1. In small bowl or cup, briefly beat egg until nearly uniform in color.

2. Add remaining ingredients and mix well to combine.

3. Spray microwave-safe plate with nonstick cooking spray.

4. Pour batter onto plate and spread into a 7- to 8-inch circle.

5. Microwave on high for 2 minutes.

6. Remove from oven and flip over to allow bottom to dry a little. Cool.

Flatbreads, Tortillas, and Pizza Crusts

Flatbread

(cornmeal)

MAKES 1 FLATBREAD

Imagine soft flatbread, not quite as flat as a tortilla.
This flatbread is understated in flavor and very pretty in form and color.

1 egg

1 tablespoon canola oil

1 tablespoon applesauce

$\frac{1}{16}$ teaspoon salt

$2\frac{1}{2}$ tablespoons cornmeal

$\frac{1}{2}$ teaspoon baking powder

Baked on: microwave-safe dinner plate

1. In small bowl or cup, briefly beat egg until nearly uniform in color.

2. Add remaining ingredients and mix well to combine.

3. Spray microwave-safe plate with nonstick cooking spray.

4. Pour batter onto plate and spread into a 7- to 8-inch circle.

5. Microwave on high for 2 minutes.

6. Remove from oven and flip over to allow bottom to dry a little. Cool.

Flatbread

(sorghum flour)
MAKES 1 FLATBREAD

Gather your favorite fillings for a quick lunch! This flatbread is thicker than a tortilla, but thinner than a slice of bread and soft and pliable.

1 egg

2 teaspoons canola oil

1 tablespoon applesauce

1/16 teaspoon salt

2 tablespoons sorghum flour

1/2 teaspoon baking powder

1/8 teaspoon sugar

Baked on: microwave-safe dinner plate

1. In small bowl or cup, briefly beat egg until nearly uniform in color.

2. Add remaining ingredients and mix well to combine.

3. Spray microwave-safe plate with nonstick cooking spray.

4. Pour batter onto plate and spread into a 7- to 8-inch circle.

5. Microwave on high for 2 minutes.

6. Remove from oven and flip over to allow bottom to dry a little. Cool.

Flatbreads, Tortillas, and Pizza Crusts

Flour Tortilla

(brown rice flour)
MAKES 1 TORTILLA

*A flat, dry, flour tortilla that's plain in flavor
and perfect for soft tacos, sandwich wraps, and fajitas.*

1 egg

1/16 teaspoon salt

2 tablespoons brown rice flour

1/8 teaspoon sugar

Baked on: microwave-safe dinner plate

1. In small bowl or cup, briefly beat egg until frothy (with varying bubble sizes).

2. Add remaining ingredients and mix well to combine.

3. Spray microwave-safe plate with nonstick cooking spray.

4. Pour batter onto plate and spread into a 7- to 8-inch circle.

5. Microwave on high for 2 minutes.

6. Remove from oven and flip over to allow bottom to dry a little. Cool.

Flour Tortilla

(cornmeal)

MAKES 1 TORTILLA

A pliable, very flat tortilla with a pleasant corn taste.

1 egg

1/16 teaspoon salt

2 1/2 tablespoons cornmeal

1/4 teaspoon sugar

Baked on: microwave-safe dinner plate

1. In small bowl or cup, briefly beat egg until frothy (with varying bubble sizes).
2. Add remaining ingredients and mix well to combine.
3. Spray microwave-safe plate with nonstick cooking spray.
4. Pour batter onto plate and spread into a 7- to 8-inch circle.
5. Microwave on high for 2 minutes.
6. Remove from oven and flip over to allow bottom to dry a little. Cool.

Flour Tortilla

(sorghum flour)
MAKES 1 TORTILLA

This is a very flavorful tortilla with full-grain taste!

1 egg

1/16 teaspoon salt

2 tablespoons sorghum flour

1/4 teaspoon sugar

Baked on: microwave-safe dinner plate

1. In small bowl or cup, briefly beat egg until frothy (with varying bubble sizes).
2. Add remaining ingredients and mix well to combine.
3. Spray microwave-safe plate with nonstick cooking spray.
4. Pour batter onto plate and spread into a 7- to 8-inch circle.
5. Microwave on high for 2 minutes.
6. Remove from oven and flip over to allow bottom to dry a little. Cool.

Pizza Crust

(brown rice flour)
MAKES A 6-INCH INDIVIDUAL CRUST

This is a super-fast pizza crust—less than two minutes in the microwave. The crust crisps nicely once topped and finished in a toaster oven or traditional oven.

1 egg

2 teaspoons canola oil

2 tablespoons applesauce

1/16 teaspoon salt

3 tablespoons brown rice flour

1/2 teaspoon baking powder

Baked on: microwave-safe round plate

1. In small bowl or cup, briefly beat egg until nearly uniform in color.
2. Add remaining ingredients and mix well to combine. The dough will look like a creamy paste.
3. Spray microwave-safe plate with nonstick cooking spray.
4. Spread batter into a 6-inch circle.
5. Microwave on high for 1 minute and 30 seconds.
6. Remove from plate and cool.
7. Place crust on metal tray or foil, top with your favorite toppings.
8. Finish baking in toaster oven (or conventional oven) at 400°F until cheese is melted and crust is crisp. Baking time will be approximately 8 to 10 minutes.

Note for Pizza Crusts: Although these pizza crusts have good taste and form, their texture is not quite as chewy as I prefer in a pizza crust. If you like a chewy crust and should you have xanthan gum in your pantry, I suggest you add 1/4 teaspoon of xanthan gum to the recipe at the same time the flour is added.

Flatbreads, Tortillas, and Pizza Crusts

Pizza Crust

(cornmeal)
MAKES A 6-INCH INDIVIDUAL CRUST

The cornmeal makes this thin pizza crust a little unconventional.
The crust is somewhat gritty in texture (in an understated way)
and mild in flavor. I think you will enjoy it!

1 egg

2 teaspoons canola oil

1 tablespoon applesauce

1/16 teaspoon salt

3½ tablespoons cornmeal

½ teaspoon baking powder

Baked on: microwave-safe round plate

1. In small bowl or cup, briefly beat egg until nearly uniform in color.

2. Add remaining ingredients and mix well to combine. The dough will look like a creamy paste.

3. Spray microwave-safe plate with nonstick cooking spray.

4. Spread batter into a 6-inch circle.

5. Microwave on high for 1 minute and 30 seconds.

6. Remove from plate and cool.

7. Place crust on metal tray or foil, top with your favorite toppings.

8. Finish baking in toaster oven (or conventional oven) at 400°F until cheese is melted and crust is crisp. Baking time will be approximately 8 to 10 minutes.

Pizza Crust

(sorghum flour)
MAKES A 6-INCH INDIVIDUAL CRUST

This dough is a little difficult to spread into a circle.
Using the back of a spoon helps tremendously! At 6 inches in diameter
this crust is medium-thick. Spread thinner for a crispier pizza.

1 egg

2 teaspoons canola oil

1 tablespoon applesauce

1/16 teaspoon salt

3 tablespoons sorghum flour

1/2 teaspoon baking powder

Baked on: microwave-safe round plate

1. In small bowl or cup, briefly beat egg until nearly uniform in color.

2. Add remaining ingredients and mix well to combine. The dough will look like a creamy paste.

3. Spray microwave-safe plate with nonstick cooking spray.

4. Spread batter into a 6-inch circle.

5. Microwave on high for 1 minute and 30 seconds.

6. Remove from plate and cool.

7. Place crust on metal tray or foil, top with your favorite toppings.

8. Finish baking in toaster oven (or conventional oven) at 400°F until cheese is melted and crust is crisp. Baking time will be approximately 8 to 10 minutes.

Flatbreads, Tortillas, and Pizza Crusts

CHAPTER 6

Sides

In this chapter you will find an eclectic mix of gluten-free side dishes that you probably never dreamed of making using your microwave. Whether steaming an ear of corn in the husk or creating traditional potato salad, you're likely to be amazed. The most incredible of all, for the die-hard foodies among us, is the Hollandaise Sauce that doesn't separate after standing. I hope you try this decadent sauce over your favorite vegetables or fish, or better yet, as part of the Eggs Florentine recipe on page 15.

Corn on the Cob

SERVES 1

This may be one of the easiest recipes in history. It is my favorite way to make corn on the cob—no mess, no fuss, easier shucking, and "steamed" to perfection. I like mine without salt or butter—it is that good.

1 ear of corn, unshucked

sprinkling of salt and pat of
    butter (optional)

1. Cut off tuft of silks at the top of the ear of corn.
2. Cut off the stem base of corn if very long.
3. Place unshucked ear of corn in microwave.
4. Microwave on high for 3 minutes.
5. Corn will be VERY hot. Carefully remove husks.
6. Top with salt and butter if desired.

Corn Pudding

(cornmeal)
SERVES 2

Not quite a custard, not quite a bread, this pudding is an old-fashioned and delicious side dish, perfect with baked chicken, meatloaf, or other homey entree! After the pudding is baked, I like to sprinkle a little freshly ground pepper on top.

1 egg

1 tablespoon canola oil

¼ cup plain lowfat yogurt

1/16 teaspoon salt

⅛ teaspoon baking powder

1 teaspoon cornmeal

1 teaspoon sugar

⅓ cup frozen corn

freshly ground pepper (optional)

Baked in: 2-cup ramekin or other straight-sided microwave-safe bowl

1. In small bowl or cup, briefly beat egg until almost uniform in color.
2. Add remaining ingredients, except corn, and mix well to combine.
3. Add corn and mix well.
4. Spray 2-cup ramekin with nonstick cooking spray.
5. Pour batter into ramekin and tap base to level batter.
6. Microwave on high for 2 minutes.
7. Serve warm with freshly ground pepper on top if desired.

German Potato Salad

I love this potato salad! If you are even more pressed for time, you can substitute 2 tablespoons Italian salad dressing (be sure it is gluten-free) for the salt, water, apple cider vinegar, and parsley. Hot or cold, this potato salad is great with almost any meal. The parsley makes the salad prettier, but it's not critical to this recipe.

1 medium white or red potato (6 ounces; 170 grams)

1½ tablespoons finely chopped onion

⅛ teaspoon salt

1 tablespoon water

1 tablespoon apple cider vinegar

pinch of dried parsley

1. Wash potato and pierce several times with a fork (to allow steam to escape).

2. Microwave on high for 2½ minutes, or until potato is tender.

3. Carefully peel potato, if desired, and cut into thin slices.

4. Place in small bowl.

5. Add remaining ingredients and mix well, but gently.

6. Refrigerate until ready to serve.

Hard-Boiled Egg

SERVES 1

A traditional hard-boiled egg doesn't do so well in a microwave. However, using a poaching technique, you get a perfectly cooked egg that can be chopped for egg salad or added to potato salad. A slightly overcooked egg in the microwave can pop. Please use caution when handling the hot egg and water!

1 cup water

1 egg

1. In 2-cup microwave-safe bowl or cup, microwave water on high for 1½ minutes, or until boiling.

2. Crack egg into boiling water and microwave on high for 1 minute and 20 seconds.

3. Carefully remove hard boiled egg and discard any frothy bits.

Hollandaise Sauce

SERVES 2

A rich, traditional hollandaise sauce in just about a minute.
It's not particularly a diet food, but it's delicious over eggs, chicken, or vegetables.
This version is rich in lemon flavor. For milder flavor, reduce the lemon juice
to 2 teaspoons and thin with a teaspoon or so of water if needed.

1 egg yolk

¼ cup butter, softened

1 tablespoon lemon juice

1. Place all ingredients in microwave-safe cup.
2. Stir well to combine.
3. Microwave on high for four 10-second intervals, mixing the ingredients very well every 10 seconds.
4. Serve hot.

Note: Butter is easily softened in the microwave by placing it in a microwave-safe dish and cooking on high for 5 to 10 seconds.

Portobello for Sandwich

MAKES 1

My daughter got me hooked on these beautiful mushrooms.
She enjoys her portobello alone as the "burger" while I like mine on top of a burger.
Portobello mushrooms are tender in just 2 minutes and firm like meat.

1 large portobello mushroom cap (1½ to 2 ounces; 60 grams)

1 teaspoon olive oil

scant ¹⁄₁₆ teaspoon garlic salt

1. Wash and dry mushroom.

2. Remove and discard stem.

3. Place bottom-side up on microwave-safe plate.

4. Sprinkle with olive oil and garlic salt.

5. Microwave on high for 2 minutes.

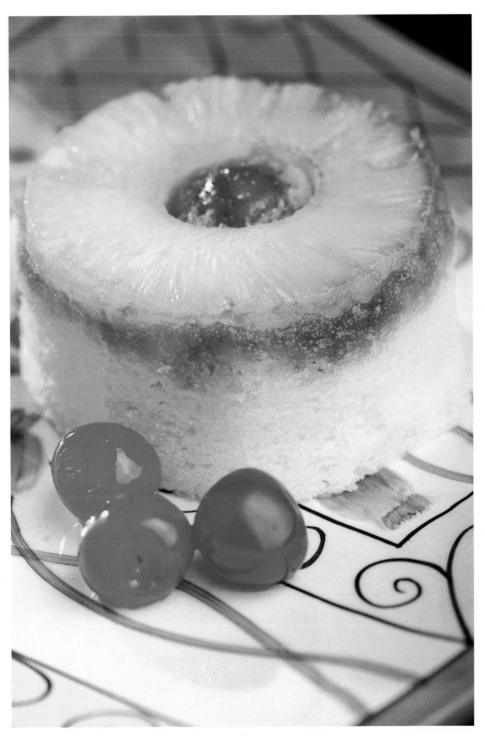

Pineapple Upside Down Cake, white rice flour, page 108

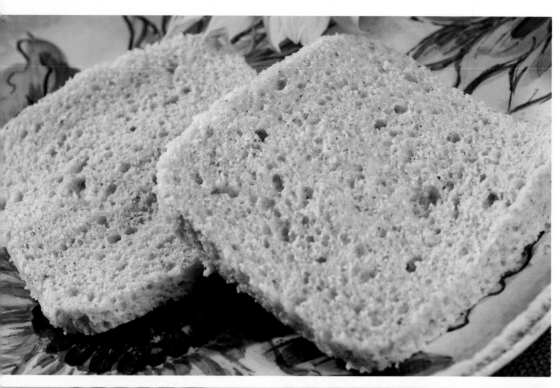

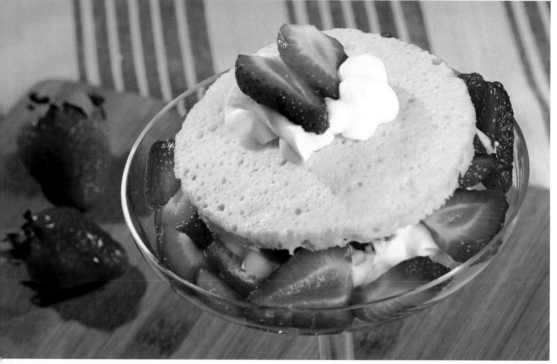

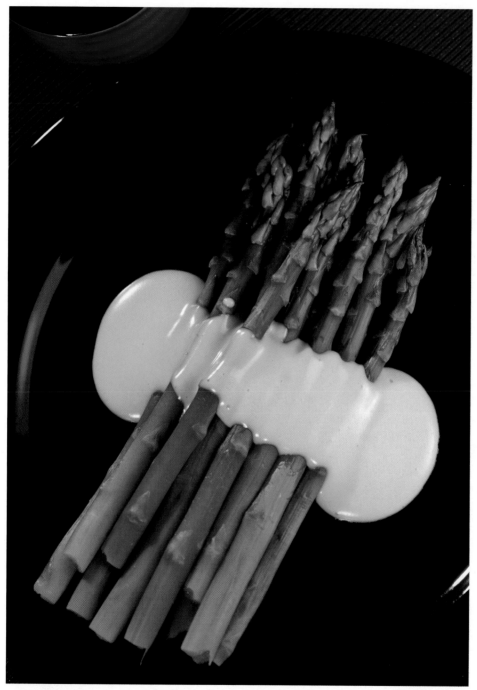

Hollandaise Sauce, page 73 (above); Sandwich Bread, sorghum flour, page 33 (facing page, top); Strawberry shortcake using Chiffon Cake, brown rice flour, page 80 (facing page, bottom)

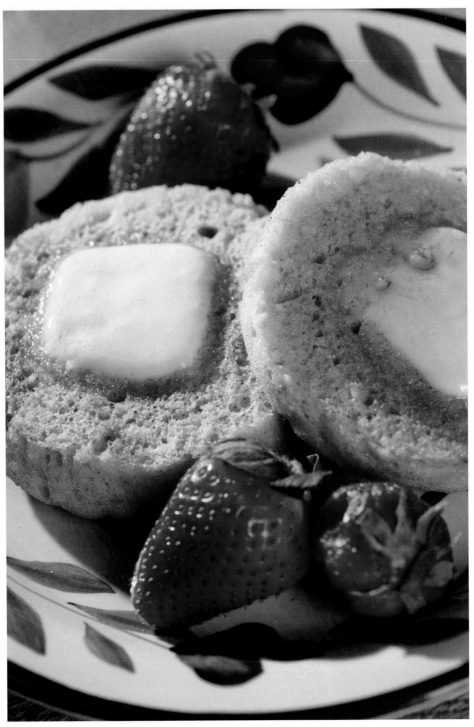

English Muffin, brown rice flour, page 16

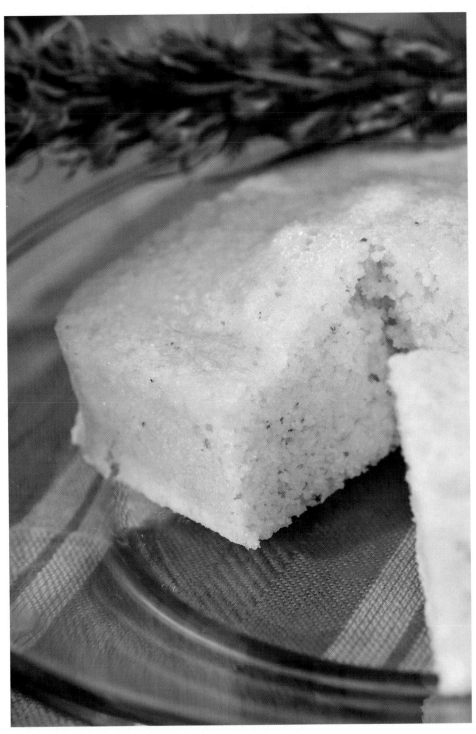

Cornbread (cornmeal), page 28

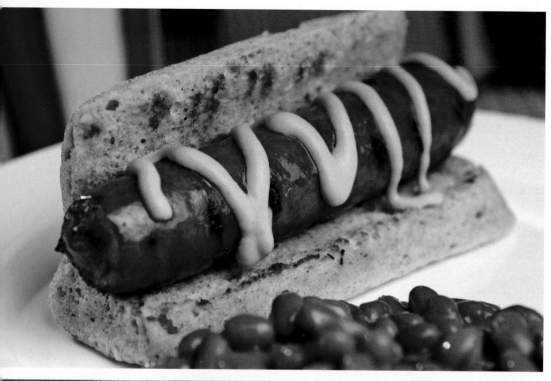

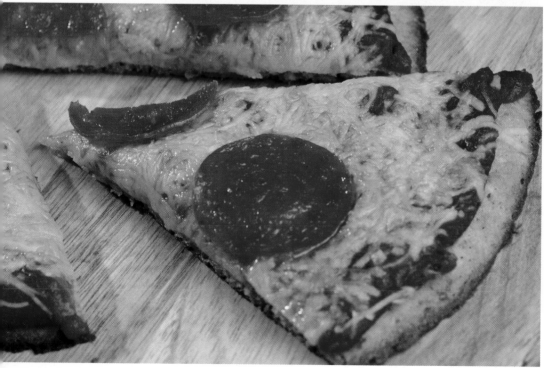

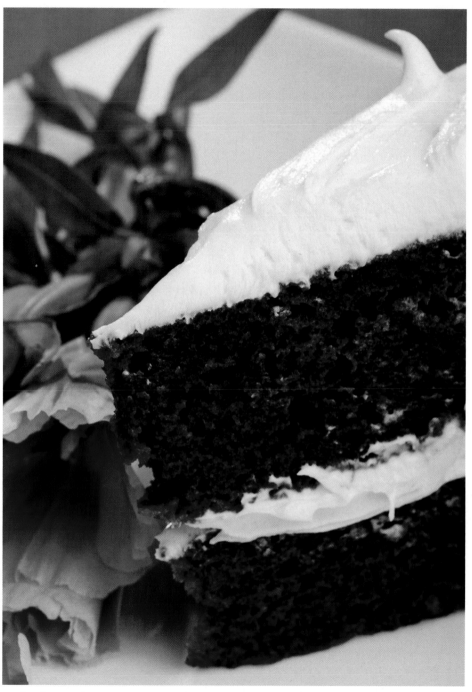

Red Velvet Cake, brown rice flour, page 110 (above); Hot Dog Roll, sorghum flour, page 43 (facing page, top); Pizza Crust, sorghum flour, page 65 (facing page, bottom)

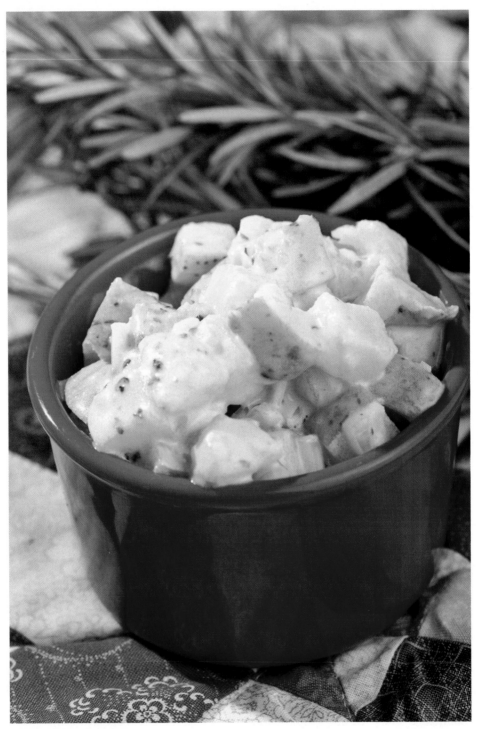

Potato Salad, page 75

Potato Salad

SERVES 1

*This is a quick, traditional potato salad that is so easy to make!
White, red, or Yukon gold potatoes are all good choices for this recipe
(Russet potatoes are not a great choice because they may fall apart).
I don't peel my potato, but you can if you prefer. Please be sure to read
the label to ensure your choice of Italian salad dressing is gluten-free.*

1 medium white or red potato
(6 ounces; 170 grams)

1½ teaspoons finely chopped
onion

1½ tablespoons mayonnaise

sprinkle of salt and pepper

1 tablespoon Italian salad
dressing

½ hard-boiled egg, chopped
(optional)

pinch of parsley (for color)

1. Wash potato and pierce several
   times with a fork (to allow steam
   to escape).

2. Microwave on high for 2½ minutes,
   or until potato is tender.

3. Carefully peel potato, if desired, and
   cut into small cubes.

4. Add remaining ingredients and mix
   well, but gently.

5. Refrigerate until ready to serve.

Stuffed Mushrooms

MAKES 3 MUSHROOMS

So, everyone is eating great appetizers and you're supposed to just sit by and smile? Well, here's a fast and quick solution: scrumptious stuffed mushrooms. Enjoy! I know I did while testing them!

3 medium mushrooms
  (3 to 3½ ounces; 100 grams)

1 fully cooked sausage link,
  minced

1 tablespoon minced onion

1 teaspoon mayonnaise

1. Wash and dry mushrooms.
2. Remove stems and set tops (bottoms up) aside on microwave-safe plate.
3. Finely chop stems of mushrooms and place in small bowl.
4. Add remaining ingredients and mix well.
5. Place mixture in mushroom tops.
6. Microwave on high for 2 minutes.

Note: Be sure to read the ingredients on your sausage. Many are gluten-free, but not all.

CHAPTER 7

Yellow Cakes and White Cakes

It may be hard to believe, but you can create nearly any kind of cake in the microwave.

Without taking the time to beat egg whites to stiff peaks, you can have angel food cake, chiffon cake, and sponge cake. Although these cakes normally require beating the eggs to stiff peaks, it is not necessary for any recipe in this book. Amazing! Or, how about a perfect traditional cake to celebrate a birthday?

Note: The foam-based cakes in this book will rise considerably, then settle, leaving the cake with perfect texture. Sometimes that settling will be perfectly straight, sometimes a little lopsided. This will not affect the taste in the slightest! It is interesting to note that the addition of just a little water makes for a moister sponge cake.

Whatever the occasion, I hope a special cake makes it complete. Life shouldn't be about food, yet good food can make life better!

And for icing on the cake, look to Chapter 10 or to the premade icings in your local grocery store. Remember to read the label!

Angel Food Cake

(brown rice flour)
SERVES 1

This might be one of the most amazing recipes in this book! You don't even have to beat the egg whites to peaks. The flavor and texture are true to the original!

2 egg whites

2 teaspoons brown rice flour

½ teaspoon baking powder

1 tablespoon sugar

⅛ teaspoon water

3 drops vanilla

Baked in: 2-cup ramekin or other straight-sided microwave-safe bowl

1. In small bowl or cup, briefly beat egg whites to small frothy bubbles.
2. Add remaining ingredients and mix well to fully combine.
3. Spray 2-cup ramekin with nonstick cooking spray.
4. Pour batter into ramekin and tap base to level batter.
5. Microwave on high for 2 minutes. Cake will rise considerably and then settle during baking.
6. Gently remove from dish and cool.

Chiffon Cake

(brown rice flour)
SERVES 1

A chiffon cake is spongy like an angel food cake or sponge cake, but richer because fat is added. Like a sponge cake, it uses whole eggs. Really, it tastes like a cross between a sponge cake and a traditional squishy cake!

1 egg

2 teaspoons brown rice flour

½ teaspoon baking powder

1 tablespoon sugar

1 teaspoon canola oil

3 drops vanilla

Baked in: 2-cup ramekin or other straight-sided microwave-safe bowl

1. In small bowl or cup, briefly beat egg until nearly uniform in color.

2. Add remaining ingredients and mix well to fully combine.

3. Spray 2-cup ramekin with nonstick cooking spray.

4. Pour batter into ramekin and tap base to level batter.

5. Microwave on high for 1 minute and 45 seconds. Cake will rise and then settle during baking.

6. Gently remove from dish and cool.

Lemon Cake

(brown rice flour)
SERVES 2

*This moist, delicately flavored cake is made from
whole grain, and it's one of my favorites!*

1 egg

1 tablespoon plus 1 teaspoon
canola oil

3 tablespoons plain lowfat
yogurt

1/16 teaspoon salt

3 tablespoons brown rice flour

1/2 teaspoon baking powder

2 tablespoons sugar

2 teaspoons lemon juice

Baked in: 2-cup ramekin or other
straight-sided microwave-safe bowl

1. In small bowl or cup, briefly beat egg
   until almost uniform in color.

2. Add remaining ingredients and mix
   well to combine.

3. Spray 2-cup ramekin with nonstick
   cooking spray.

4. Pour batter into ramekin and tap
   base to level batter.

5. Microwave on high for 2 minutes.
   Cake will rise and then settle a little
   during baking.

6. Gently remove from dish and cool.

7. Ice as desired.

Lemon Poppy Seed Pound Cake

(brown rice flour)
SERVES 2

This is likely my most favorite pound cake. The poppy seeds
may be omitted, but their bright nutty flavor is tasty!

1 egg

1 tablespoon plus 1 teaspoon
canola oil

2½ tablespoons applesauce

1/16 teaspoon salt

3 tablespoons brown rice flour

⅛ teaspoon baking powder

1 tablespoon plus 1 teaspoon
sugar

2 teaspoons lemon juice

½ teaspoon poppy seeds

LEMON GLAZE (OPTIONAL):

1 teaspoon lemon juice

1 teaspoon milk or cream

3 tablespoons confectioner's
sugar

Baked in: 2-cup ramekin or other
straight-sided microwave-safe bowl

1. In small bowl or cup, briefly beat egg
   until almost uniform in color.

2. Add remaining ingredients and mix
   well to combine.

3. Spray 2-cup ramekin with nonstick
   cooking spray.

4. Pour batter into ramekin and tap
   base to level batter.

5. Microwave on high for 2 minutes.
   Cake will rise and then settle a little
   during baking.

6. Gently remove from dish and cool.

7. For glaze, combine all glaze ingredients in small cup.

8. Mix well to combine, then pour over
   cooled cake.

Pound Cake

(brown rice flour)
SERVES 2

This is a traditional vanilla pound cake. It has a tight crumb
with a few wayward larger holes and is moist and very tasty.

1 egg

1 tablespoon plus 1 teaspoon
  canola oil

3 tablespoons applesauce

$\frac{1}{16}$ teaspoon salt

3 tablespoons brown rice flour

$\frac{1}{8}$ teaspoon baking powder

1 tablespoon plus 1 teaspoon
  sugar

$\frac{1}{8}$ teaspoon vanilla

Baked in: 2-cup ramekin or other straight-sided microwave-safe bowl

1. In small bowl or cup, briefly beat egg until almost uniform in color.

2. Add remaining ingredients and mix well to combine.

3. Spray 2-cup ramekin with nonstick cooking spray.

4. Pour batter into ramekin and tap base to level batter.

5. Microwave on high for 2 minutes. Cake will rise and then settle a little during baking.

6. Gently remove from dish and cool.

Yellow Cakes and White Cakes

Sponge Cake

(brown rice flour)
SERVES 1

A sponge cake is a lot like an angel food cake, except it is made with whole eggs. Both are spongy in texture. This recipe makes a beautiful sponge cake, ready to be adorned with fruit, ice cream, or enjoyed plain. This cake is also among the prettiest of the sponge-type cakes in this book!

1 egg

2 teaspoons brown rice flour

½ teaspoon baking powder

1 tablespoon sugar

¼ teaspoon water

3 drops vanilla

Baked in: 2-cup ramekin or other straight-sided microwave-safe bowl

1. In small bowl or cup, briefly beat egg until nearly uniform in color.

2. Add remaining ingredients and mix well to fully combine.

3. Spray 2-cup ramekin with nonstick cooking spray.

4. Pour batter into ramekin and tap base to level batter.

5. Microwave on high for 1 minute and 45 seconds. Cake will rise and then settle during baking.

6. Gently remove from dish and cool.

White Cake

(white rice flour)
SERVES 2

This cake is not beautiful, but it's dead-on in flavor and texture. I apologize for making you use half of an egg white, but repeated formulations showed there was just no alternative. To measure, whisk the egg white slightly and measure out 1 tablespoon plus 1 teaspoon to equal ½ egg white. (Or you can just eyeball it!)

1½ egg whites

1 tablespoon canola oil

3 tablespoons plain lowfat yogurt

⅟16 teaspoon salt

2½ tablespoons white rice flour

½ teaspoon baking powder

2 tablespoons sugar

⅛ teaspoon vanilla

Baked in: 2-cup ramekin or other straight-sided microwave-safe bowl

1. In small bowl or cup, beat egg whites well.

2. Add remaining ingredients and mix well to combine.

3. Spray 2-cup ramekin with nonstick cooking spray.

4. Pour batter into ramekin and tap base to level batter.

5. Microwave on high for 2 minutes. Cake will rise and then settle a little during baking.

6. Gently remove from dish and cool.

7. Ice as desired.

Yellow Cake

(white rice flour)
SERVES 2

Soft and squishy, this cake is a winner!
Increase the sugar to 2 tablespoons if you want a really sweet cake.

1 egg

1 tablespoon plus 1 teaspoon canola oil

3 tablespoons plain lowfat yogurt

1/16 teaspoon salt

2 1/2 tablespoons white rice flour

1/2 teaspoon baking powder

1 1/2 tablespoons sugar

1/8 teaspoon vanilla

Baked in: 2-cup ramekin or other straight-sided microwave-safe bowl

1. In small bowl or cup, briefly beat egg until almost uniform in color.

2. Add remaining ingredients and mix well to combine.

3. Spray 2-cup ramekin with nonstick cooking spray.

4. Pour batter into ramekin and tap base to level batter.

5. Microwave on high for 2 minutes. Cake will rise and then settle a little during baking.

6. Gently remove from dish and cool.

7. Ice as desired.

Yellow Torte Cake

(white rice flour)
SERVES 2

*This is an eggy cake, inspired by an English multilayered cake.
It is perfect for slicing in half and layering with whipped cream, pudding,
and fruit. Presentation is everything when it comes to this cake!*

1 egg

1 tablespoon canola oil

3 tablespoons plain lowfat
  yogurt

1/16 teaspoon salt

1 1/2 tablespoons white rice flour

1/2 teaspoon baking powder

1 1/2 tablespoons sugar

1/8 teaspoon vanilla

Baked in: 2-cup ramekin or other straight-sided microwave-safe bowl

1. In small bowl or cup, briefly beat egg until almost uniform in color.

2. Add remaining ingredients and mix well to combine.

3. Spray 2-cup ramekin with nonstick cooking spray.

4. Pour batter into ramekin and tap base to level batter.

5. Microwave on high for 2 minutes. Cake will rise and then settle a little during baking.

6. Gently remove from dish and cool.

7. Slice cake horizontally and fill with whipped cream, pudding, and fruit as desired.

Note: For a great strawberry shortcake, place 2 tablespoons vanilla yogurt in between 2 layers, and place sliced strawberries on top of the yogurt and on top of the cake.

CHAPTER 8

Chocolate Cakes

I have so many favorites in this chapter! There is a springy sponge cake, a squishy traditional-style cake, and a dense pound cake with a tight crumb. And, if you have no gluten-free flours on hand, you can still make the Extreme Chocolate Cake, which is both delicate and full of chocolate flavor. Any of the traditional-style cakes would be enhanced with an icing from Chapter 10—or a premade icing from your local market. Please remember to check the ingredient labels!

I want to point out that only one cake in this chapter must be eaten the day that it is made: the cornstarch version of Chocolate Cake. It is also the only cornstarch-based cake in this book. The flavor is good and the texture is great, but, unlike brown rice, white rice, and sorghum, cornstarch does not hold its moist texture overnight. For that reason, cornstarch is almost never used alone in this book. To those of you who are longtime gluten-free bakers, it may seem odd that "grittier" flours hold moisture better in these recipes—however, it's true!

Chocolate Angel Food Cake

(brown rice flour)
SERVES 1

*This cake has a subtle chocolate flavor. Although it's great alone,
pairing it with raspberries and a little melted jam would be a wonderful treat.
For even more chocolate flavor, a half teaspoon of cocoa may be added
in place of the same amount of brown rice flour.*

2 egg whites

2 teaspoons brown rice flour

¼ teaspoon baking powder

1 tablespoon sugar

2 teaspoons chocolate syrup

Baked in: 2-cup ramekin or other straight-sided microwave-safe bowl

1. In small bowl or cup, briefly beat egg whites to small frothy bubbles.
2. Add remaining ingredients and mix well to fully combine.
3. Spray 2-cup ramekin with nonstick cooking spray.
4. Pour batter into ramekin and tap base to level batter.
5. Microwave on high for 2 minutes. Cake will rise considerably and then settle during baking.
6. Gently remove from dish and cool.

Chocolate Cake

(brown rice flour)
SERVES 2

Need to calm that craving for dark chocolate flavor?
This is the cake for you!

1 egg

1½ tablespoons canola oil

3 tablespoons applesauce

¹⁄₁₆ teaspoon salt

1½ tablespoons brown rice flour

1 tablespoon plus 1 teaspoon cocoa

⅛ teaspoon baking soda

1 tablespoon sugar

⅛ teaspoon vanilla

Baked in: 2-cup ramekin or other straight-sided microwave-safe bowl

1. In small bowl or cup, briefly beat egg until almost uniform in color.
2. Add remaining ingredients and mix well to combine.
3. Spray 2-cup ramekin with nonstick cooking spray.
4. Pour batter into ramekin and tap base to level batter.
5. Microwave on high for 2 minutes. Cake will rise and then settle a little during baking.
6. Gently remove from dish and cool.
7. Ice as desired.

Chocolate Cake

(cornstarch)
SERVES 2

*This cake bakes up very, very moist, but is just right after cooling. It has a
slightly tighter crumb than the other two versions. It is not too sweet, so if you
want that supersweet, from-the-box taste, increase the sugar just a little.
As mentioned in the chapter introduction, this cake should be eaten same day.*

1 egg

1½ tablespoons canola oil

3 tablespoons applesauce

¹⁄₁₆ teaspoon salt

2½ tablespoons cornstarch

1 tablespoon plus 1 teaspoon
cocoa

½ teaspoon baking powder

1 tablespoon sugar

⅛ teaspoon vanilla

Baked in: 2-cup ramekin or other
straight-sided microwave-safe bowl

1. In small bowl or cup, briefly beat egg
   until almost uniform in color.

2. Add remaining ingredients and mix
   well to combine.

3. Spray 2-cup ramekin with nonstick
   cooking spray.

4. Pour batter into ramekin and tap
   base to level batter.

5. Microwave on high for 2 minutes.
   Cake will rise and then settle a little
   during baking.

6. Gently remove from dish and cool.

7. Ice as desired.

Chocolate Cake

(sorghum flour)
SERVES 2

*This recipe makes a single layer petite cake
that is perfect for two light eaters or one with the munchies!*

1 egg

2 tablespoons canola oil

3 tablespoons applesauce

$\frac{1}{16}$ teaspoon salt

2 tablespoons sorghum flour

1 tablespoon plus 1 teaspoon cocoa

$\frac{1}{8}$ teaspoon baking soda

1 tablespoon sugar

$\frac{1}{8}$ teaspoon vanilla

Baked in: 2-cup ramekin or other straight-sided microwave-safe bowl

1. In small bowl or cup, briefly beat egg until almost uniform in color.
2. Add remaining ingredients and mix well to combine.
3. Spray 2-cup ramekin with nonstick cooking spray.
4. Pour batter into ramekin and tap base to level batter.
5. Microwave on high for 2 minutes Cake will rise and then settle a little during baking.
6. Gently remove from dish and cool.
7. Ice as desired.

Chocolate Cake Roll

(brown rice flour)
SERVES 2

*The cake roll is a flat sponge cake topped with whipped cream
or other filling, such as pudding or jam, and rolled into a log.*

1 egg

2 teaspoons brown rice flour

¼ teaspoon baking powder

1 tablespoon sugar

2 teaspoons chocolate syrup

FILLING:

¼ cup whipped cream or
  pudding

Baked on: large microwave-safe plate

1. In small bowl or cup, briefly beat egg
   until nearly uniform in color.

2. Add remaining ingredients and mix
   well to fully combine.

3. Spray microwave-safe plate with
   nonstick cooking spray.

4. Pour batter to form a square of
   about 6 inches.

5. Microwave on high for 1 minute and
   45 seconds. Cake will be approximately ¼- to ⅓-inch in thickness.

6. Gently remove from plate and cool.

7. As soon as the cake is cool, turn it
   upside down on plate. (Cake will
   begin to crack if left to cool for
   a longer period of time.)

8. Spread filling over cake, leaving a bit
   of edge bare.

9. Roll into a log.

Chocolate Pound Cake

(brown rice flour)
SERVES 2

This cake is denser with a tighter crumb than a traditional cake.
Just a dusting of confectioner's sugar would be wonderful on top.

1 egg

1 tablespoon canola oil

3 tablespoons applesauce

1/16 teaspoon salt

2 tablespoons brown rice flour

1 tablespoon plus 1 teaspoon cocoa

1/8 teaspoon baking powder

1 tablespoon plus 1 teaspoon sugar

1/8 teaspoon vanilla

TOPPING (OPTIONAL):

1 teaspoon confectioner's sugar

Baked in: 2-cup ramekin or other straight-sided microwave-safe bowl

1. In small bowl or cup, briefly beat egg until almost uniform in color.

2. Add remaining ingredients and mix well to combine.

3. Spray 2-cup ramekin with nonstick cooking spray.

4. Pour batter into ramekin and tap base to level batter.

5. Microwave on high for 2 minutes. Cake will rise and then settle a little during baking.

6. Gently remove from dish and cool.

7. Dust with confectioner's sugar if desired.

Chocolate Pound Cake

(sorghum flour)
SERVES 2

This pound cake is dense with an extremely tight crumb.
Plain or adorned with fruit and ice cream, this cake is just plain good.

1 egg

1½ tablespoons canola oil

3 tablespoons applesauce

¹⁄₁₆ teaspoon salt

2½ tablespoons sorghum flour

1 tablespoon plus 1 teaspoon cocoa

⅛ teaspoon baking powder

1 tablespoon plus 1 teaspoon sugar

⅛ teaspoon vanilla

Baked in: 2-cup ramekin or other straight-sided microwave-safe bowl

1. In small bowl or cup, briefly beat egg until almost uniform in color.

2. Add remaining ingredients and mix well to combine.

3. Spray 2-cup ramekin with nonstick cooking spray.

4. Pour batter into ramekin and tap base to level batter.

5. Microwave on high for 2 minutes. Cake will rise and then settle a little during baking.

6. Gently remove from dish and cool.

Chocolate Sponge Cake

(brown rice flour)
SERVES 1

The chocolate counterpart of traditional sponge cake.
A drizzle of chocolate and fresh berries would be delicious here!
This cake tastes like hot chocolate in spongy form—a good thing.

1 egg

1 teaspoon brown rice flour

1 teaspoon cocoa

½ teaspoon baking powder

1 tablespoon sugar

¼ teaspoon water

3 drops vanilla

Baked in: 2-cup ramekin or other straight-sided microwave-safe bowl

1. In small bowl or cup, briefly beat egg until nearly uniform in color.
2. Add remaining ingredients and mix well to fully combine.
3. Spray 2-cup ramekin with nonstick cooking spray.
4. Pour batter into ramekin and tap base to level batter.
5. Microwave on high for 1 minute and 45 seconds. Cake will rise and then settle during baking.
6. Gently remove from dish and cool.

Extreme Chocolate Cake

SERVES 2

By using cocoa as the flour, you will have a very delicate cake with extreme chocolate flavor. Pair it with the Chocolate Ganache recipe on page 115 for true decadence. This cake received two thumbs up from my dear friend Maddie!

1 egg

1½ tablespoons canola oil

3 tablespoons applesauce

¹⁄₁₆ teaspoon salt

2½ tablespoons cocoa

⅛ teaspoon baking soda

1 tablespoon sugar

⅛ teaspoon vanilla

Baked in: 2-cup ramekin or other straight-sided microwave-safe bowl

1. In small bowl or cup, briefly beat egg until almost uniform in color.

2. Add remaining ingredients and mix well to combine.

3. Spray 2-cup ramekin with nonstick cooking spray.

4. Pour batter into ramekin and tap base to level batter.

5. Microwave on high for 2 minutes. Cake will rise and then settle a little during baking.

6. Gently remove from dish and cool.

7. Ice as desired.

CHAPTER 9

Other Cakes

This chapter contains quite the assortment of cakes! If I had to choose my favorite, it would be the Marble Cake. It has a great balance of chocolate and vanilla flavor. My second favorite is the Red Velvet Cake—either version. Whether store-bought or made from a recipe in Chapter 10, a little icing would be delicious on these cakes!

I suggest that you do not freeze either version of the Carrot Cake. Freezing distorts the color of the carrots. Instead, enjoy them on the day you make them.

Banana Cake

(white rice flour)
SERVES 2

Banana cake is my friend Diane's favorite.
Unlike banana bread, this cake is very light!

1 egg

1 tablespoon plus 1 teaspoon canola oil

¼ cup baby food banana (Beech-Nut Stage 2)

1/16 teaspoon salt

2½ tablespoons white rice flour

½ teaspoon baking powder

1 tablespoon sugar

⅛ teaspoon vanilla

Baked in: 2-cup ramekin or other straight-sided microwave-safe bowl

1. In small bowl or cup, briefly beat egg until almost uniform in color.

2. Add remaining ingredients and mix well to combine.

3. Spray 2-cup ramekin with nonstick cooking spray.

4. Pour batter into ramekin and tap base to level batter.

5. Microwave on high for 2 minutes. Cake will rise and then settle a little during baking.

6. Gently remove from dish and cool.

7. Ice as desired.

Carrot Cake

(brown rice flour)
SERVES 2

*This carrot cake is slightly lighter in texture
than the sorghum version but equally as good!*

1 egg

1 tablespoon plus 1 teaspoon canola oil

2 tablespoons applesauce

1/16 teaspoon salt

2 1/2 tablespoons brown rice flour

1/3 cup packed, grated carrots

1/8 teaspoon baking soda

1 1/2 tablespoons brown sugar

2 tablespoons chopped pecans

2 tablespoons raisins, chopped

1/8 teaspoon pumpkin pie spice

Baked in: 2-cup ramekin or other straight-sided microwave-safe bowl

1. In small bowl or cup, briefly beat egg until almost uniform in color.

2. Add remaining ingredients and mix well to combine.

3. Spray 2-cup ramekin with nonstick cooking spray.

4. Pour batter into ramekin and tap base to level batter.

5. Microwave on high for 2 minutes. Cake will rise and then settle a little during baking.

6. Gently remove from dish and cool.

7. Ice as desired.

Carrot Cake

(sorghum flour)
SERVES 2

This cake is delicious alone
or frosted with cream cheese icing.

1 egg

1½ tablespoons canola oil

2 tablespoons applesauce

⅟₁₆ teaspoon salt

3 tablespoons sorghum flour

⅓ cup packed, grated carrots

⅛ teaspoon baking soda

1½ tablespoons brown sugar

2 tablespoons chopped pecans

2 tablespoons raisins, chopped

⅛ teaspoon pumpkin pie spice

Baked in: 2-cup ramekin or other straight-sided microwave-safe bowl

1. In small bowl or cup, briefly beat egg until almost uniform in color.

2. Add remaining ingredients and mix well to combine.

3. Spray 2-cup ramekin with nonstick cooking spray.

4. Pour batter into ramekin and tap base to level batter.

5. Microwave on high for 2 minutes. Cake will rise and then settle a little during baking.

6. Gently remove from dish and cool.

7. Ice as desired.

Marble Cake

(brown rice flour)
SERVES 2

This cake is a flavorful marble cake. And so very easy.
The use of chocolate syrup could not work better!

1 egg

1 tablespoon plus 1 teaspoon
    canola oil

3 tablespoons plain lowfat
    yogurt

1/16 teaspoon salt

3 tablespoons brown rice flour

1/2 teaspoon baking powder

1 1/2 tablespoons sugar

1/8 teaspoon vanilla

2 teaspoons chocolate syrup

Baked in: 2-cup ramekin or other straight-sided microwave-safe bowl

1. In small bowl or cup, briefly beat egg until almost uniform in color.
2. Add remaining ingredients, except chocolate syrup, and mix well to combine.
3. Spray 2-cup ramekin with nonstick cooking spray.
4. Pour batter into ramekin and tap base to level batter.
5. Drizzle chocolate syrup over top of batter and "cut" in a swirl pattern with the edge of a knife.
6. Microwave on high for 2 minutes. Cake will rise and then settle a little during baking.
7. Gently remove from dish and cool.
8. Ice as desired.

Orange Valencia Cake

(brown rice flour)
SERVES 2

This cake was inspired by the gluten-free cake that was once
available at Starbucks. Hopefully, you will like this version even better!
Enjoy this soft, dense, moist cake at room temperature.

1 egg

1 tablespoon plus 1 teaspoon
   canola oil

2 tablespoons frozen orange
   juice concentrate

1 tablespoon applesauce

$\frac{1}{16}$ teaspoon salt

3 tablespoons brown rice flour

$\frac{1}{8}$ teaspoon baking powder

1 tablespoon sugar

3 drops vanilla

Baked in: 2-cup ramekin or other
straight-sided microwave-safe bowl

1. In small bowl or cup, briefly beat egg
   until almost uniform in color.

2. Add remaining ingredients and mix
   well to combine.

3. Spray 2-cup ramekin with nonstick
   cooking spray.

4. Pour batter into ramekin and tap
   base to level batter.

5. Microwave on high for 2 minutes.
   Cake will rise and then settle a little
   during baking.

6. Gently remove from dish and cool.

Pineapple Upside Down Cake

(white rice flour)
SERVES 2

This recipe uses the white rice flour version of Yellow Cake poured atop a brown sugar and pineapple base. Then it is inverted after baking.

1 egg

1 tablespoon plus 1 teaspoon canola oil

3 tablespoons plain lowfat yogurt

1/16 teaspoon salt

2½ tablespoons white rice flour

½ teaspoon baking powder

1½ tablespoons sugar

⅛ teaspoon vanilla

BASE:

1 pineapple slice

1 tablespoon brown sugar (dark preferred)

1 maraschino cherry or several raisins

Baked in: 2-cup ramekin or other straight-sided microwave-safe bowl

1. Prepare the base.

2. Spray a 2-cup ramekin with nonstick cooking spray.

3. Place pineapple slice, brown sugar, and cherry or raisins in the bottom of the prepared ramekin. Set aside.

4. In small bowl or cup, briefly beat egg until almost uniform in color.

5. Add remaining ingredients and mix well to combine.

6. Pour batter over prepared base and tap ramekin to level batter.

7. Microwave on high for 2 minutes. Cake will rise and then settle a little during baking.

8. Gently remove from dish, invert, and cool.

Pumpkin Cake Roll

(brown rice flour)
SERVES 2

By making this cake with baby food squash or sweet potatoes, you can avoid opening an entire can of pumpkin. The flavor is very much the same. Enjoy your own private pumpkin cake roll with cream cheese icing as the filling. Lucky you!

1 egg

2 teaspoons brown rice flour

¼ teaspoon baking powder

1 tablespoon sugar

1 tablespoon baby food squash or sweet potatoes (Beech-Nut Stage 2)

⅛ teaspoon pumpkin pie spice

FILLING:

½ recipe Cream Cheese Icing on page 117

TOPPING:

1 teaspoon confectioner's sugar

Baked on: large microwave-safe plate

1. In small bowl or cup, briefly beat egg to small frothy bubbles.

2. Add remaining ingredients and mix well to fully combine.

3. Spray microwave-safe plate with nonstick cooking spray.

4. Pour batter into a 5-inch square.

5. Microwave on high for 1 minute and 45 seconds. Cake will be approximately ¼- to ⅓-inch in thickness.

6. Gently remove from plate and cool.

7. As soon as cake is cool turn it upside down on the plate. (Cake will begin to crack if left to cool for a longer period of time.)

8. Spread filling over cake, leaving a bit of edge bare.

9. Roll into a log.

10. Dust top with confectioner's sugar.

Other Cakes

Red Velvet Cake

(brown rice flour)
SERVES 2

*Red velvet cake has a texture somewhere between that of
a traditional squishy cake and a pound cake. While the cake is
not chocolate, cocoa is the basis of the underlying flavor. Enjoy!*

1 egg

1 tablespoon plus 1 teaspoon canola oil

3 tablespoons applesauce

$1/16$ teaspoon salt

$2\frac{1}{2}$ tablespoons brown rice flour

1 teaspoon cocoa

$1/8$ teaspoon baking powder

$1/8$ teaspoon baking soda

1 tablespoon plus 1 teaspoon sugar

$1/8$ teaspoon vanilla

$1/4$ teaspoon red food coloring

Baked in: 2-cup ramekin or other straight-sided microwave-safe bowl

1. In small bowl or cup, briefly beat egg until almost uniform in color.

2. Add remaining ingredients and mix well to combine.

3. Spray 2-cup ramekin with nonstick cooking spray.

4. Pour batter into ramekin and tap base to level batter.

5. Microwave on high for 2 minutes. Cake will rise and then settle a little during baking.

6. Gently remove from dish and cool.

Red Velvet Cake

(sorghum flour)
SERVES 2

This cake is very much like the traditional red velvet cake.
Please note that during baking, it will rise very high and then settle again.
The end result is just right.

1 egg

1½ tablespoons canola oil

3 tablespoons applesauce

1/16 teaspoon salt

3 tablespoons sorghum flour

1 teaspoon cocoa

1/8 teaspoon baking powder

1/8 teaspoon baking soda

1 tablespoon plus 1 teaspoon sugar

1/8 teaspoon vanilla

1/4 teaspoon red food coloring

Baked in: 2-cup ramekin or other straight-sided microwave-safe bowl

1. In small bowl or cup, briefly beat egg until almost uniform in color.
2. Add remaining ingredients and mix well to combine.
3. Spray 2-cup ramekin with nonstick cooking spray.
4. Pour batter into ramekin and tap base to level batter.
5. Microwave on high for 2 minutes. Cake will rise and then settle during baking.
6. Gently remove from dish and cool.

Spice Cake

(brown rice flour)
SERVES 2

I've used pumpkin pie spice to avoid tiny measurements of multiple spices.
This cake is soft and squishy with a light spice flavor.
For robust flavor, double the amount of pumpkin pie spice.

1 egg

1 tablespoon plus 1 teaspoon canola oil

3 tablespoons plain lowfat yogurt

1/16 teaspoon salt

2 tablespoons plus 2 teaspoons brown rice flour

1/2 teaspoon baking powder

1 1/2 tablespoons sugar

1/8 teaspoon vanilla

1/8 teaspoon pumpkin pie spice

Baked in: 2-cup ramekin or other straight-sided microwave-safe bowl

1. In small bowl or cup, briefly beat egg until almost uniform in color.

2. Add remaining ingredients and mix well to combine.

3. Spray 2-cup ramekin with nonstick cooking spray.

4. Pour batter into ramekin and tap base to level batter.

5. Microwave on high for 2 minutes. Cake will rise and then settle a little during baking.

6. Gently remove from dish and cool.

7. Ice as desired.

Icings

Many traditional, store-bought icings are gluten-free. However, the cakes in this book need no more than ½ cup of icing. So, I've included a few icing recipes that are quick and easy to prepare.

To avoid prolonged beating, which cuts the raw sugar taste in homemade icings, I briefly microwave the ingredients in many recipes. Although this may sound odd, it makes a notable difference.

I also use a regular, single-size Hershey's milk chocolate bar in several of these recipes. The bar weighs 43 grams and is available at the checkout in most grocery stores!

Chocolate Ganache

SERVES 2

This is a thick ganache that is perfect to pour over any chocolate, yellow, or white cake. It is not too sweet but rather luxurious in flavor!

½ **Hershey's milk chocolate bar**

1 tablespoon sour cream

1. In small microwave-safe bowl or cup, place chocolate bar and sour cream.
2. Microwave on high for 10 seconds. Stir.
3. Microwave for another 10 seconds. Stir until creamy.
4. Spread over top of cake and allow to drip down the sides.

Chocolate Icing

MAKES APPROXIMATELY ½ CUP

A traditional chocolate icing.

1 cup confectioner's sugar

2 teaspoons milk or cream

½ Hershey's milk chocolate bar, broken into pieces

2 tablespoons butter, cut into cubes

1. Combine all ingredients in microwave-safe small cup.

2. Stir together.

3. Microwave on high for 30 seconds to soften butter.

4. Beat (by hand) until smooth and creamy.

5. If icing is a bit warm, allow to cool. Then spread over cooled cake.

Cream Cheese Icing

MAKES APPROXIMATELY ½ CUP

Unlike the other icing recipes in this book, this icing is not prepared using a microwave. (Note: Microwaving severely damages the texture of this icing.) Instead, a smooth, creamy icing is achieved by hand mixing it until smooth.

1 cup confectioner's sugar

2 teaspoons milk

3 tablespoons cream cheese

3 drops vanilla

1. Combine all ingredients in small cup.
2. Stir together.
3. Beat (by hand) until smooth and creamy.
4. Spread over cooled cake.

Lemon Glaze

MAKES APPROXIMATELY 2 TABLESPOONS

1 teaspoon lemon juice

1 teaspoon milk or cream

3 tablespoons confectioner's sugar

1. Combine all ingredients in small cup.

2. Mix well, then pour over cooled cake.

Note: For a vanilla glaze, replace the lemon juice with ¼ teaspoon vanilla and add an additional ¾ teaspoon milk.

Lemon Icing

MAKES APPROXIMATELY ½ CUP

A traditional lemon icing.

1 cup confectioner's sugar

1 teaspoon lemon juice

2 tablespoons butter, cut into cubes

1. Combine all ingredients in small cup.

2. Microwave on high for 30 seconds to soften butter.

3. Beat (by hand) until smooth and creamy.

4. If icing is a bit warm, allow to cool. Then spread over cooled cake.

Peanut Butter Icing

MAKES APPROXIMATELY ½ CUP

This is my favorite icing. I love it on chocolate cake!

1 cup confectioner's sugar

2 teaspoons milk or cream

1 tablespoon butter, cut into cubes

1 tablespoon peanut butter

3 drops vanilla

1. Combine all ingredients in small cup.
2. Stir together.
3. Microwave on high for 15 seconds to soften butter.
4. Beat (by hand) until smooth and creamy.
5. If icing is a bit warm, allow to cool. Then spread over cooled cake.

Note: If the cooking time in step 3 is increased to 35 seconds, the icing will have a fondant consistency, which is just plain cool.

Vanilla Icing

MAKES APPROXIMATELY ½ CUP

A traditional vanilla icing.

1 cup confectioner's sugar

1½ teaspoons milk or cream

2 tablespoons butter, cut into cubes

4 drops vanilla

1. Combine all ingredients in small cup.
2. Stir together.
3. Microwave on high for 30 seconds to soften butter.
4. Beat (by hand) until smooth and creamy.
5. If icing is a bit warm, allow to cool. Then spread over cooled cake.

Snack Cakes and Cookies

I like the idea of pulling a warm brownie out of the microwave, putting a scoop of ice cream on it, and drizzling chocolate syrup on top. In just a few quick minutes, the person with the "special" diet is just another person enjoying a treat.

One of my favorite recipes in this chapter is the Peanut Butter Bars, sorghum flour version. If you like peanut butter, I hope you'll try it!

Brownie

(brown rice flour)
MAKES 2

Sweet, soft, and moist. Allow the brownie to cool
for several minutes for best texture!

1 egg

1 tablespoon canola oil

1 tablespoon applesauce

$\frac{1}{16}$ teaspoon salt

1 tablespoon brown rice flour

1 tablespoon cocoa

2 tablespoons sugar

$\frac{1}{8}$ teaspoon vanilla

Baked in: 2-cup ramekin or other straight-sided microwave-safe bowl

1. In small bowl or cup, briefly beat egg until almost uniform in color.

2. Add remaining ingredients and mix well to combine.

3. Spray 2-cup ramekin with nonstick cooking spray.

4. Pour batter into ramekin and tap base to level batter.

5. Microwave on high for 2 minutes.

6. Gently remove from dish and cool.

Brownie

(sorghum flour)
MAKES 2

This brownie has more of the chewiness that is typical of traditional brownies.
One could say that it has more overall brownie mouthfeel.
Simply put, it was preferred among our taste testers.

1 egg

1 tablespoon canola oil

1 tablespoon applesauce

1/16 teaspoon salt

1 tablespoon and 1 teaspoon
sorghum flour

1 tablespoon cocoa

2 tablespoons sugar

1/8 teaspoon vanilla

Baked in: 2-cup ramekin or other straight-sided microwave-safe bowl

1. In small bowl or cup, briefly beat egg until almost uniform in color.
2. Add remaining ingredients and mix well to combine.
3. Spray 2-cup ramekin with nonstick cooking spray.
4. Pour batter into ramekin and tap base to level batter.
5. Microwave on high for 2 minutes.
6. Gently remove from dish and cool.

Butterscotch Krimpet-style Snack Cake

(brown rice flour)
SERVES 1

I had a difficult time locating the flavoring for this snack cake, until I found LorAnn flavoring oils at the pharmacy counter! How strange is that? LorAnn flavoring oils are also available online (see the Appendix). I hope you enjoy this gluten-free version of my very favorite snacking cake!

1 egg

1½ teaspoons canola oil

2 teaspoons brown rice flour

½ teaspoon baking powder

1 tablespoon sugar

¼ teaspoon water

2 drops LorAnn butterscotch flavor oil

ICING:

3 tablespoons confectioner's sugar

1 teaspoon shortening

2 drops LorAnn butterscotch flavor oil

¾ teaspoon milk

Baked in: 2-cup square ramekin or other straight-sided microwave-safe bowl

1. In small bowl or cup, briefly beat egg until nearly uniform in color.

2. Add remaining ingredients and mix well to fully combine.

3. Spray 2-cup ramekin with nonstick cooking spray.

4. Pour batter into ramekin and tap base to level batter.

5. Microwave on high for 1 minute and 45 seconds. Cake will rise and then settle during baking.

6. Gently remove from dish and cool.

7. Combine all icing ingredients in small cup and beat until smooth.

8. Spread over top of snack cake.

9. Cut cake into thirds to form three krimpets.

Chocolate Chip Cookie Bars

(brown rice flour)
SERVES 2

This is a delicious cookie bar. When mixing, you will find the batter
very thin. When eating, you will find great moist texture.

1 egg

1 tablespoon canola oil

1 tablespoon applesauce

$\frac{1}{16}$ teaspoon salt

2 tablespoons brown rice flour

2 tablespoons brown sugar

$\frac{1}{8}$ teaspoon vanilla

2 tablespoons chocolate chips, chopped

Baked in: 2-cup ramekin or other straight-sided microwave-safe bowl

1. In small bowl or cup, briefly beat egg until almost uniform in color.
2. Add remaining ingredients, except chocolate chips, and mix well to combine.
3. Fold in chocolate chips.
4. Spray 2-cup ramekin with nonstick cooking spray.
5. Pour batter into ramekin and tap base to level batter.
6. Microwave on high for 2 minutes.
7. Gently remove from dish and cool.

Chocolate Chip Cookie Bars

(sorghum flour)
SERVES 2

I first tried making these cookies with whole semi-sweet chocolate chips, but the batter was too thin to support them. So, I simply chopped the chips well and voilà, a great cookie bar.

1 egg

1 tablespoon canola oil

1 tablespoon applesauce

1/16 teaspoon salt

2 tablespoons and 1 teaspoon cocoa

2 tablespoons sugar

1/8 teaspoon vanilla

2 tablespoons chocolate chips, chopped

Baked in: 2-cup ramekin or other straight-sided microwave-safe bowl

1. In small bowl or cup, briefly beat egg until almost uniform in color.
2. Add remaining ingredients, except chocolate chips, and mix well to combine.
3. Fold in chocolate chips.
4. Spray 2-cup ramekin with nonstick cooking spray.
5. Pour batter into ramekin and tap base to level batter.
6. Microwave on high for 2 minutes.
7. Gently remove from dish and cool.

Snack Cakes and Cookies

Crispy Rice Treat

MAKES 1

Although I love an entire pan of these treats,
this recipe provides a treat with portion control.

½ tablespoon butter

3 large marshmallows

¾ cup gluten-free crispy rice cereal

1. In small microwave-safe cup or bowl, combine butter and marshmallows.

2. Microwave for approximately 30 seconds, until quite melted.

3. Stir well.

4. Add cereal and stir well to combine.

5. Spray ramekin or other small serving dish with nonstick spray.

6. Press mixture into ramekin and cool.

Gingerbread

(brown rice flour or white rice flour)
SERVES 2

*I suggest using dark brown sugar in this recipe if you have it.
It provides a slightly darker color, which just seems right. Despite the
seemingly large amount of ginger, this is a mildly spiced gingerbread.
Although I prefer my gingerbread without icing, the vanilla icing in
Chapter 10 would be a nice addition if you have a sweet tooth.*

1 egg

1 tablespoon canola oil

2½ tablespoons applesauce

1/16 teaspoon salt

3 tablespoons plus 1 teaspoon
brown or white rice flour

½ teaspoon baking powder

1 tablespoon brown sugar

¼ teaspoon ginger

⅛ teaspoon cinnamon

Baked in: 2-cup ramekin or other
straight-sided microwave-safe bowl

1. In small bowl or cup, briefly beat egg
until almost uniform in color.

2. Add remaining ingredients and mix
well to combine.

3. Spray 2-cup ramekin with nonstick
cooking spray.

4. Pour batter into ramekin and tap
base to level batter.

5. Microwave on high for 2 minutes.
Bread will rise and then settle a little
during baking.

6. Gently remove from dish and cool.

7. Ice as desired.

Oatmeal Snacking Cake

(brown rice flour)
SERVES 2

This recipe is based upon a very old oatmeal cake recipe. It needs no adornment, though it is very good with cream cheese or vanilla icing (see Chapter 10).

1 egg

1 tablespoon plus 1 teaspoon canola oil

3 tablespoons applesauce

1/16 teaspoon salt

2 tablespoons brown rice flour

1/4 cup gluten-free oatmeal

1/8 teaspoon baking soda

1 1/2 tablespoons brown sugar

2 tablespoons raisins, chopped

2 tablespoons chopped pecans

1/4 teaspoon pumpkin pie spice

Baked in: 2-cup ramekin or other straight-sided microwave-safe bowl

1. In small bowl or cup, briefly beat egg until almost uniform in color.

2. Add remaining ingredients and mix well to combine.

3. Spray 2-cup ramekin with nonstick cooking spray.

4. Pour batter into ramekin and tap base to level batter.

5. Microwave on high for 2 minutes. Cake will rise and then settle a little during baking.

6. Gently remove from dish and cool.

7. Ice as desired.

Oatmeal Snacking Cake

(sorghum flour)
SERVES 2

I normally pair regular sugar with sorghum, but here I opted for brown sugar for a fuller flavored cake. Nuts would be a nice addition if you like.

1 egg

1½ tablespoons canola oil

3 tablespoons applesauce

rounded ¹⁄₁₆ teaspoon salt

2½ tablespoons sorghum flour

¼ cup gluten-free oatmeal

½ teaspoon baking powder

1½ tablespoons brown sugar

2 tablespoons mini chocolate chips

2 tablespoons chopped pecans (optional)

⅛ teaspoon vanilla

Baked in: 2-cup ramekin or other straight-sided microwave-safe bowl

1. In small bowl or cup, briefly beat egg until almost uniform in color.

2. Add remaining ingredients and mix well to combine.

3. Spray 2-cup ramekin with nonstick cooking spray.

4. Pour batter into ramekin and tap base to level batter.

5. Microwave on high for 2 minutes. Cake will rise and then settle a little during baking.

6. Gently remove from dish and cool.

Peanut Butter Bars

(brown rice flour)
SERVES 2

If you are a peanut butter fan, you will like this cookie bar!
The chocolate chips melt into an awesome topping.

1 egg

2 teaspoons canola oil

1 tablespoon applesauce

$\frac{1}{16}$ teaspoon salt

1 tablespoon brown rice flour

1$\frac{1}{2}$ tablespoons peanut butter

2 tablespoons sugar

$\frac{1}{8}$ teaspoon vanilla

TOPPING:

2 tablespoons mini chocolate
   chips

Baked in: 2-cup ramekin or other straight-sided microwave-safe bowl

1. In small bowl or cup, briefly beat egg until almost uniform in color.

2. Add remaining ingredients and mix well to combine.

3. Spray 2-cup ramekin with nonstick cooking spray.

4. Pour batter into ramekin and tap base to level batter.

5. Microwave on high for 2 minutes.

6. Immediately sprinkle 2 tablespoons of mini chocolate chips on top and allow to melt (melts faster if covered), then spread.

7. Gently remove from dish and cool.

Peanut Butter Bars

(sorghum flour)
SERVES 2

*These bars have lots of good peanut butter flavor and
are a bit chewy. The chocolate layer on top is just right.*

1 egg

2 teaspoons canola oil

1 tablespoon applesauce

1/16 teaspoon salt

1 tablespoon plus 1 teaspoon
sorghum flour

1½ tablespoons peanut butter

2 tablespoons sugar

1/8 teaspoon vanilla

TOPPING:

2 tablespoons mini chocolate
chips

Baked in: 2-cup ramekin or other
straight-sided microwave-safe bowl

1. In small bowl or cup, briefly beat egg
until almost uniform in color.

2. Add remaining ingredients and mix
well to combine.

3. Spray 2-cup ramekin with nonstick
cooking spray.

4. Pour batter into ramekin and tap
base to level batter.

5. Microwave on high for 2 minutes.

6. Immediately sprinkle 2 tablespoons
of mini chocolate chips on top
and allow to melt (melts faster if
covered), then spread.

7. Gently remove from dish and cool.

White Chocolate Chip Cookie Bars

(brown rice flour)
SERVES 2

This cookie bar offers a dense, cakey base topped with
white chocolate chips and nuts. These are addictive.

1 egg

1 tablespoon canola oil

1 tablespoon applesauce

$\frac{1}{16}$ teaspoon salt

2 tablespoons brown rice flour

2 tablespoons sugar

$\frac{1}{8}$ teaspoon vanilla

2 tablespoons white chocolate chips, chopped fine

1 tablespoon finely chopped pecans (optional)

Baked in: 2-cup ramekin or other straight-sided microwave-safe bowl

1. In small bowl or cup, briefly beat egg until almost uniform in color.
2. Add remaining ingredients, except chocolate chips and pecans, and mix well to combine.
3. Spray 2-cup ramekin with nonstick cooking spray.
4. Pour batter into ramekin and tap base to level batter.
5. Sprinkle chips and pecans on top.
6. Microwave on high for 2 minutes.
7. Gently remove from dish and cool.

CHAPTER 12

Quick Breads and Muffins

This chapter has long-time favorite quick breads and muffins. From Applesauce Bread to Blueberry Muffins, you can count on great taste, moistness, and texture. These recipes are not overly sweet as some commercial products can be.

It is my opinion that quick breads and muffins are not supposed to have the same texture or sweetness of cakes. They are a little coarser and less sugary. And that makes these the perfect addition to any meal or outing.

Applesauce Bread

(brown rice flour or white rice flour)
SERVES 2

This bread has a soft apple undertone with mild cinnamon flavor. If you have no cinnamon on hand, add a bit of vanilla to soften the flavor. The apple flavor is a bit stronger if using white rice flour. This recipe is among my favorites.

1 egg

1 tablespoon canola oil

3 tablespoons applesauce

1/16 teaspoon salt

3 tablespoons brown rice flour or 2½ tablespoons white rice flour

½ teaspoon baking powder

1 tablespoon sugar

⅛ teaspoon cinnamon

Baked in: 2-cup ramekin or other straight-sided microwave-safe bowl

1. In small bowl or cup, briefly beat egg until almost uniform in color.

2. Add remaining ingredients and mix well to combine.

3. Spray 2-cup ramekin with nonstick cooking spray.

4. Pour batter into ramekin and tap base to level batter.

5. Microwave on high for 2 minutes. Bread will rise and then settle a little during baking.

6. Gently remove from dish and cool.

Note: A sprinkling of cinnamon on top makes this quick bread prettier.

Quick Breads and Muffins

Applesauce Snacking Cake

(sorghum flour)

SERVES 2

This recipe is a feel-good, almost guilt-free treat! The raisins are chopped fine so that they don't sink to the bottom of the cake. The vanilla extract softens the whole-grain flavor of the sorghum. And the cinnamon adds a bit of spice! Vanilla icing (Chapter 10) may be added if desired.

1 egg

1 tablespoon canola oil

3 tablespoons applesauce

1/16 teaspoon salt

3½ tablespoons sorghum flour

scant ½ teaspoon baking powder

1 tablespoon sugar

1 tablespoon raisins, finely chopped

1 tablespoon nuts, finely chopped (optional)

⅛ teaspoon cinnamon

⅛ teaspoon vanilla

Baked in: 2-cup ramekin or other straight-sided microwave-safe bowl

1. In small bowl or cup, briefly beat egg until almost uniform in color.
2. Add remaining ingredients and mix well to combine.
3. Spray 2-cup ramekin with nonstick cooking spray.
4. Pour batter into ramekin and tap base to level batter.
5. Microwave on high for 2 minutes. Cake will rise and then settle a little during baking.
6. Gently remove from dish and cool.
7. Ice as desired.

Banana Bread

(brown rice flour or white rice flour)
SERVES 2

This recipe has mild banana flavor and is not too sweet.
If using brown rice flour, be sure to add the vanilla to soften its flavor.
Or, use white rice flour for more prominent banana flavor.

1 egg

1 tablespoon canola oil

3 tablespoons banana baby food (Beech-Nut Stage 2)

$\frac{1}{16}$ teaspoon salt

3 tablespoons brown rice flour or $2\frac{1}{2}$ tablespoons white rice flour

$\frac{1}{2}$ teaspoon baking powder

1 tablespoon sugar

$\frac{1}{8}$ teaspoon vanilla (optional)

Baked in: 2-cup ramekin or other straight-sided microwave-safe bowl

1. In small bowl or cup, briefly beat egg until almost uniform in color.

2. Add remaining ingredients and mix well to combine.

3. Spray 2-cup ramekin with nonstick cooking spray.

4. Pour batter into ramekin and tap base to level batter.

5. Microwave on high for 2 minutes. Bread will rise and then settle a little during baking.

6. Gently remove from dish and cool.

Quick Breads and Muffins

Banana Bread

(sorghum flour)
SERVES 2

This is a soft, sweet banana bread. A little whole-grain
flavor is there, but the flavor of the banana comes through.

1 egg

1 tablespoon canola oil

3 tablespoons banana baby
food (Beech-Nut Stage 2)

1/16 teaspoon salt

3½ tablespoons sorghum flour

½ teaspoon baking powder

1 tablespoon sugar

⅛ teaspoon vanilla (optional)

Baked in: 2-cup ramekin or other
straight-sided microwave-safe bowl

1. In small bowl or cup, briefly beat egg
   until almost uniform in color.

2. Add remaining ingredients and mix
   well to combine.

3. Spray 2-cup ramekin with nonstick
   cooking spray.

4. Pour batter into ramekin and tap
   base to level batter.

5. Microwave on high for 2 minutes.
   Bread will rise and then settle a little
   during baking.

6. Gently remove from dish and cool.

Blueberry Muffins

(brown rice flour)
MAKES 2 MUFFINS

This recipe uses plain lowfat yogurt for its thicker consistency rather than for flavor. It is the thickness of the batter that keeps the berries somewhat suspended. This muffin is pretty, very soft, a little pale in color, and bright in blueberry flavor!

1 egg

1 tablespoon canola oil

3 tablespoons plain lowfat yogurt

1/16 teaspoon salt

3 tablespoons brown rice flour

1/2 teaspoon baking powder

1 1/2 tablespoons sugar

1/8 teaspoon vanilla

1/2 cup fresh blueberries (smaller are better!)

Baked in: two 1-cup ramekins or other straight-sided microwave-safe bowls or cups

1. In small bowl or cup, briefly beat egg until almost uniform in color.

2. Add remaining ingredients, except blueberries, and mix well to combine.

3. Gently fold in blueberries.

4. Spray 1-cup ramekins with nonstick cooking spray.

5. Pour batter into ramekins and tap base of each to level batter.

6. Microwave on high for 2 minutes. Muffins will rise and then settle a little during baking.

7. Gently remove from dishes and cool.

Blueberry Muffins

(sorghum flour)
MAKES 2 MUFFINS

This recipe tastes like a slightly whole-grain version of a traditional blueberry muffin. It is very moist! Please note that these muffins take a little longer in the microwave than some of the other recipes in this book.

1 egg

1 tablespoon canola oil

3 tablespoons applesauce

1/16 teaspoon salt

scant 4 tablespoons sorghum flour

1/2 teaspoon baking powder

1 1/2 tablespoons sugar

1/8 teaspoon vanilla

1/2 cup fresh blueberries, chopped

Baked in: two 1-cup ramekins or other straight-sided microwave-safe bowls or cups

1. In small bowl or cup, briefly beat egg until almost uniform in color.
2. Add remaining ingredients, except blueberries, and mix well to combine.
3. Gently fold in blueberries.
4. Spray ramekins with nonstick cooking spray.
5. Pour batter into ramekins and tap base of each to level batter.
6. Microwave on high for 2 minutes and 30 seconds. Muffins will rise and then settle a little during baking.
7. Gently remove from dishes and cool.

Chocolate Chip Muffins

(brown rice flour)
MAKES 2 MUFFINS

The batter for these muffins is rather thin for suspending the chocolate chips, so add them on the top of the batter allowing them to sink into the batter as it bakes. These muffins have great flavor.

1 egg

1 tablespoon canola oil

3 tablespoons applesauce

1/16 teaspoon salt

3 tablespoons brown rice flour

1/8 teaspoon baking soda

1 1/2 tablespoons brown sugar

1/8 teaspoon vanilla

2 tablespoons mini chocolate chips

Baked in: two 1-cup ramekins or other straight-sided microwave-safe bowls

1. In small bowl or cup, briefly beat egg until almost uniform in color.

2. Add remaining ingredients, except chocolate chips, and mix well to combine.

3. Spray ramekins with nonstick cooking spray.

4. Pour batter into ramekins and tap bases to level batter.

5. Sprinkle chocolate chips on top.

6. Microwave on high for 2 minutes. Muffins will rise and then settle a little during baking.

7. Gently remove from dishes and cool.

Chocolate Chip Muffins

(sorghum flour)
MAKES 2 MUFFINS

*This muffin is very traditional in texture
and not too sweet. Just a good muffin!*

1 egg

1 tablespoon canola oil

3 tablespoons applesauce

1/16 teaspoon salt

scant 4 tablespoons sorghum
flour

1/2 teaspoon baking powder

1 1/2 tablespoons sugar

1/8 teaspoon vanilla

2 tablespoons mini chocolate
chips

Baked in: two 1-cup ramekins or other straight-sided microwave-safe bowls

1. In small bowl or cup, briefly beat egg until almost uniform in color.

2. Add remaining ingredients, except chocolate chips, and mix well to combine.

3. Spray ramekins with nonstick cooking spray.

4. Pour batter into ramekins and tap bases to level batter.

5. Sprinkle chocolate chips on top.

6. Microwave on high for 2 minutes and 30 seconds. Muffins will rise and then settle a little during baking.

7. Gently remove from dishes and cool.

Peach Muffins

(brown rice flour)
MAKES 2 MUFFINS

The flavor of peach cobbler in a tender muffin! Substitute cinnamon
for the nutmeg if you have none. This muffin is very moist.

1 egg

1 tablespoon canola oil

3 tablespoons applesauce

1/16 teaspoon salt

3 tablespoons brown rice flour

1/2 teaspoon baking powder

1 1/2 tablespoons sugar

1/16 teaspoon nutmeg

4 drops vanilla extract

1 peach, peeled, cored, and finely chopped (1/2 cup)

Baked in: two 1-cup ramekins or other straight-sided microwave-safe bowls or cups

1. In small bowl or cup, briefly beat egg until almost uniform in color.

2. Add remaining ingredients and mix well to combine.

3. Spray ramekins with nonstick cooking spray.

4. Pour batter into ramekins and tap bases to level batter.

5. Microwave on high for 2 minutes and 15 seconds. Muffins will rise and then settle a little during baking.

6. Gently remove from dishes and cool.

Peach Muffins

(sorghum flour)
MAKES 2 MUFFINS

These muffins are brightly spiced and bursting with fresh peach flavor!
The yogurt adds a soft smoothness to the texture of the muffin, while vanilla
softens the flavor of the sorghum flour. These are very moist.

1 egg

1 tablespoon canola oil

3 tablespoons plain lowfat
   yogurt

1/16 teaspoon salt

4 tablespoons sorghum flour

1/2 teaspoon baking powder

1 1/2 tablespoons sugar

1/16 teaspoon nutmeg

1/16 teaspoon cinnamon

4 drops vanilla extract

1 peach, peeled, cored, and
   finely chopped (1/2 cup)

Baked in: two 1-cup ramekins or other straight-sided microwave-safe bowls or cups

1. In small bowl or cup, briefly beat egg until almost uniform in color.

2. Add remaining ingredients and mix well to combine.

3. Spray ramekins with nonstick cooking spray.

4. Pour batter into ramekins and tap bases to level batter.

5. Microwave on high for 3 minutes. Muffins will rise and then settle a little during baking.

6. Gently remove from dishes and cool.

Zucchini Bread

(brown rice flour)
SERVES 2

This is an absolutely delicious way to eat your vegetables.
Bring it along on a picnic or for an after-class snack.
The bread is moist and soft, but with substance.

1 egg

1 tablespoon canola oil

½ cup packed, grated zucchini or other squash

1⁄16 teaspoon salt

3 tablespoons brown rice flour

½ teaspoon baking powder

1 tablespoon plus 1 teaspoon sugar

⅛ teaspoon cinnamon

Baked in: 2-cup ramekin or other straight-sided microwave-safe bowl

1. In small bowl or cup, briefly beat egg until almost uniform in color.

2. Add remaining ingredients and mix well to combine.

3. Spray 2-cup ramekin with nonstick cooking spray.

4. Pour batter into ramekin and tap base to level batter.

5. Microwave on high for 2 minutes. Bread will rise and then settle a little during baking.

6. Gently remove from dish and cool.

Zucchini Bread

(sorghum flour)
SERVES 2

The brown-rice version (page 149) is straight-up traditional.
With a drier crumb, but lots of moistness from the zucchini, this
sorghum-based recipe is just a little different—good, but different.

1 egg

1½ tablespoons canola oil

½ cup packed, grated zucchini
or other squash

¹⁄₁₆ teaspoon salt

3½ tablespoons sorghum flour

½ teaspoon baking powder

1 tablespoon plus 1 teaspoon
sugar

⅛ teaspoon cinnamon

Baked in: 2-cup ramekin or other
straight-sided microwave-safe bowl

1. In small bowl or cup, briefly beat
   egg until almost uniform in color.

2. Add remaining ingredients and mix
   well to combine.

3. Spray 2-cup ramekin with nonstick
   cooking spray.

4. Pour batter into ramekin and tap
   base to level batter.

5. Microwave on high for 2 minutes.
   Bread will rise and then settle a little
   during baking.

6. Gently remove from dish and cool.

CHAPTER 13

Other Desserts

When you're looking for something different to curb that sweet craving, come to this chapter.

The Crepe is an unexpected surprise. It is delicate and can be filled with so many different things. Sweet or savory, you will enjoy this recipe. Or how about a crisp or a cobbler? With just a little fruit, you are in for a treat!

Apple Crisp

(brown rice flour)
SERVES 2

*This apple crisp is quite sweet with a thick apple base
and a crisp topping. Although tasty plain, a dollop of
vanilla ice cream would be a delicious addition.*

1 large Golden Delicious or
other sweet apple, peeled,
cored, and diced
(approximately 2 cups)

1 tablespoon brown sugar

1 teaspoon brown rice flour

2 tablespoons water

⅛ teaspoon cinnamon

3 drops vanilla extract

TOPPING:

10 gluten-free animal crackers
crushed or 2½ tablespoons
other crisp cookie crushed

¼ teaspoon cinnamon

1 tablespoon brown sugar

Baked in: 2-cup ramekin or other
straight-sided microwave-safe bowl

1. Place all ingredients in ramekin or
other microwave-safe bowl.

2. Stir well. Set aside.

3. In another cup or bowl, mix topping
ingredients.

4. Sprinkle topping over apple mixture.

5. Microwave on high one minute at a
time, until apples are tender—up to
4 minutes.

6. Serve warm or cold.

Other Desserts

Blueberry Cobbler

(sorghum flour)
SERVES 2

*This cobbler is made with frozen blueberries so it
can be made any time of year! The flavor is surprisingly
light given the fuller flavor of sorghum flour. A nice dessert.*

1 egg

1 tablespoon canola oil

2 tablespoons applesauce

1/16 teaspoon salt

2 1/2 tablespoons sorghum flour

2 tablespoons sugar

1/8 teaspoon vanilla

1/2 cup frozen blueberries

Baked in: 2-cup ramekin or other straight-sided microwave-safe bowl

1. In small bowl or cup, briefly beat egg until almost uniform in color.

2. Add remaining ingredients, except blueberries, and mix well to combine.

3. Spray 2-cup ramekin with nonstick cooking spray.

4. Pour batter into ramekin and tap base to level batter.

5. Sprinkle blueberries on top.

6. Microwave on high for 2 minutes and 30 seconds.

7. Serve warm or cool.

Bread Pudding, Apple

SERVES 1

I've used the Cinnamon Raisin Bread recipe in this dish, but you could use any of the bread recipes in this book in its place.

½ prepared recipe for Cinnamon Raisin Bread (pages 25–26)

½ small apple, peeled, cored, and diced

1 egg

2 teaspoons sugar

3 tablespoons milk

3 drops vanilla

Baked in: 2-cup ramekin or other straight-sided microwave-safe bowl

1. Cut prepared bread into ½-inch cubes.

2. Place in small mixing bowl.

3. Add apples. Set aside.

4. In small cup, combine egg, sugar, milk, and vanilla.

5. Mix very well.

6. Pour over bread cubes.

7. Toss gently but thoroughly to combine.

8. Spray 2-cup ramekin with nonstick cooking spray.

9. Pour bread cube mixture into ramekin.

10. Microwave on high for 2 minutes.

Other Desserts

Crepe

(brown rice flour)
MAKES 1 CREPE

Here is a perfect opportunity to make a single beautiful crepe!
Although the browning from the pan is obviously not feasible in the microwave,
the delicate, sweet, eggy texture is there. To serve, I suggest folding the crepe
around fruit or chocolate and topping with a little whipped cream.

1 egg

1 tablespoon canola oil

1 tablespoon applesauce

1/16 teaspoon salt

1 tablespoon brown rice flour

1/4 teaspoon baking powder

1 1/2 teaspoons sugar

3 drops vanilla (optional)

Baked on: microwave-safe dinner plate

1. In small bowl or cup, briefly beat egg until frothy (with varying bubble sizes).

2. Add remaining ingredients and mix well to combine.

3. Spray microwave-safe plate with nonstick cooking spray.

4. Pour batter onto plate and spread into a 5-inch circle. The crepe will spread during baking.

5. Microwave on high for 2 minutes.

6. Remove from microwave oven and flip over to allow bottom to dry a little.

Peach Cobbler

(brown rice flour)
SERVES 2

Enjoy this cobbler when the peaches are ripe and juicy.
This cobbler is not too sweet and lightly spiced.

1 egg

1 tablespoon canola oil

2 tablespoons applesauce

$\frac{1}{16}$ teaspoon salt

2 tablespoons brown rice flour

1$\frac{1}{2}$ tablespoons sugar

$\frac{1}{8}$ teaspoon vanilla

$\frac{1}{16}$ teaspoon cinnamon

1 medium peach, peeled,
   pitted, and diced
   (about $\frac{1}{2}$ cup)

Baked in: 2-cup ramekin or other straight-sided microwave-safe bowl

1. In small bowl or cup, briefly beat egg until almost uniform in color.

2. Add remaining ingredients, except peaches, and mix well to combine.

3. Spray 2-cup ramekin with nonstick cooking spray.

4. Pour batter into ramekin and tap base to level batter.

5. Sprinkle peaches on top.

6. Microwave on high for 2 minutes.

7. Serve warm or cool.

Peach Crisp

(cornstarch)

SERVES 2

I created this recipe during the heart of peach season in Maryland. If you have a good peach, this recipe will give you a great crisp! If your peach is a bit out of season, add an extra teaspoon of sugar to the peach after you chop it. I won't tell. Added spices are kept to a minimum so the peach flavor shines through.

1 large peach, peeled, pitted, and diced (approximately 1½ cups)

1 teaspoon sugar

½ teaspoon cornstarch

1 tablespoon water

1/16 teaspoon cinnamon or 1/32 teaspoon nutmeg

TOPPING:

10 gluten-free animal crackers crushed or 2½ tablespoons other crisp cookie crushed

⅛ teaspoon cinnamon or 1/16 teaspoon nutmeg

2½ teaspoons brown sugar

Baked in: 2-cup ramekin or other straight-sided microwave-safe bowl

1. Place all ingredients in ramekin or other microwave-safe bowl.

2. Stir well. Set aside.

3. In another cup or bowl, mix topping ingredients.

4. Sprinkle topping over peaches.

5. Microwave on high for 4 minutes.

6. Serve warm or cold.

Note: "Cling" peaches have flesh that clings to the pit. "Freestone" peaches have flesh that pulls away cleanly from the pit. Cling peaches usually come early in the season followed later by freestone peaches. Both are delicious.

Poached Pear

SERVES 1

An elegant dish for one.

1 medium pear, not quite ripe (a little firm)

1 tablespoon brown sugar

$\frac{1}{16}$ teaspoon cinnamon

1 teaspoon butter (thin pat)

Baked in: microwave-safe mug

1. Peel pear. Cut off blossom end to make a stable base.

2. Leaving stem intact, cut pear in half from stem to blossom end.

3. Use spoon to remove seeds.

4. Place in microwave-safe mug.

5. Sprinkle sugar, cinnamon, and bits of butter over pear.

6. Cover with plastic wrap. Pierce several holes in the plastic wrap to vent.

7. Microwave on high for 1 or 2 minutes, until pear is soft.

8. Place pear upright on serving plate and pour sauce over top.

Raspberry Cobbler

(brown rice flour)
SERVES 2

This is a traditional cobbler chock-full of berries that sink into a soft cake-like base. The bottom of the cobbler is almost creamy, but not quite.

1 egg

1 tablespoon canola oil

2 tablespoons applesauce

1/16 teaspoon salt

2 tablespoons brown rice flour

2 tablespoons sugar

1/8 teaspoon vanilla

1/2 cup fresh raspberries

Baked in: 2-cup ramekin or other straight-sided microwave-safe bowl

1. In small bowl or cup, briefly beat egg until almost uniform in color.
2. Add remaining ingredients, except raspberries, and mix well to combine.
3. Spray 2-cup ramekin with nonstick cooking spray.
4. Pour batter into ramekin and tap base to level batter.
5. Sprinkle raspberries on top.
6. Microwave on high for 2 minutes.
7. Serve warm or cool.

Rice Pudding

(cornstarch)
SERVES 2

*This recipe is so easy, it makes me wonder why
I don't make nice homemade desserts more often!*

1 egg

⅓ cup milk

1 tablespoon plus 1 teaspoon
   sugar

1 tablespoon raisins

pinch of cinnamon or nutmeg

⅛ teaspoon vanilla

½ cup cooked rice

½ teaspoon cornstarch

Baked in: microwave-safe measuring
cup or bowl

Served in: 2-cup ramekin or two 1-cup
ramekins

1. In microwave-safe bowl or large
   measuring cup (2 cups), briefly beat
   egg until almost uniform in color.

2. Add remaining ingredients and mix
   well to combine.

3. Microwave on high for 1 minute.

4. Continue to microwave for
   10-second intervals until mixture
   is almost boiling. (Do not boil
   because custard will curdle.)

5. Place into ramekin(s) and refrigerate.
   Pudding will thicken upon cooling.

Scalloped Apples

SERVES 2

Nothing is better than a side dish of scalloped apples!

1 large Golden Delicious or other sweet apple, peeled, cored, and sliced thick (2 cups)

1 tablespoon brown sugar

2 tablespoons water

⅛ teaspoon cinnamon

Baked in: 2-cup ramekin or other microwave-safe bowl

1. Place all ingredients in ramekin.

2. Stir well.

3. Cover with plastic wrap. Pierce several holes in the plastic wrap to vent.

4. Microwave on high for between 4 and 5 minutes. The bowl will be very hot!

5. Stir well.

6. Serve hot or cold.

Note: To make chunky applesauce, add one additional tablespoon of water and increase cooking time by approximately 2 minutes. Smash apples with tines of fork. Serve hot or cold.

Gluten-Free Resources

NATIONAL GLUTEN-FREE SUPPORT GROUPS

American Celiac Society

www.americanceliacsociety.org
PO Box 23455
New Orleans, LA 70183
504-737-3293

Celiac Disease Foundation

www.celiac.org
13251 Ventura Boulevard, #1
Studio City, CA 91604
818-990-2354

Celiac Sprue Association/ USA Inc.

www.csaceliacs.org
PO Box 31700
Omaha, NE 68131
877-CSA-4CSA
(877-272-4272)

The Gluten Intolerance Group of North America

www.gluten.net
31214 124th Avenue SE
Seattle, WA 98092
253-833-6655

LOCAL CELIAC SUPPORT GROUPS

Celiac.com

www.celiac.com
Scroll down the home page to locate index, then click on support groups.

GLUTEN-FREE MAIL ORDER SUPPLIERS

In this book, only a handful of specialty items are necessary. All of the ingredients used should be readily available to you at your local market or health food

163

store. Listed below are places to order the few items that may not be available locally, as well as some sources of gluten-free supplies. Note, Rumford baking powder is available from Clabber Girl, detailed below.

Allergy Grocer.com (also known as Miss Roben's)

www.allergygrocer.com

Offers a variety of gluten-free baking supplies and mixes.

Amazon.com

www.amazon.com

Amazon is a surprising home for many gluten-free foods and baking supplies, including toaster bags and the sometimes elusive square glass microwave-safe dishes for baking the bread recipes in this book! Savings are available when ordering in quantity, but be sure you like the item before you order in bulk. Many books about living gluten-free can be ordered quite reasonably there as well.

Bob's Red Mill

www.bobsredmill.com

Offers a large variety of gluten-free baking supplies and flours.

Celiac.com

www.celiac.com

Home to the "Gluten-Free Mall," which includes numerous suppliers of gluten-free foods, books, personal care products, and more.

Clabber Girl

www.clabbergirl.com

Purchase Rumford baking powder right from the source.

The Gluten-Free Pantry

www.glutenfree.com

PO Box 840

Glastonbury, CT 06033

860-633-3826

Shop this site for tons of premade, gluten-free products, condiments, pastas, and baking supplies and mixes.

Ener-G Foods

www.ener-g.com

PO Box 84487

5960 1st Avenue South

Seattle, WA 98124

800-331-5222

This site boasts "Over 150 Gluten-Free, Wheat-Free, Dairy-Free, Nut-Free, and Kosher-Certified Products!" It also offers monthly specials.

LorAnn Oils

www.Lorannoils.com
4518 Aurelius Road
Lansing, Michigan 48909
517-882-0215

These gluten-free flavorings (including the butterscotch used in this book) are 3 to 4 times stronger than grocery store extracts, so be sure when substituting that you use only ¼ to ½ teaspoon for 1 teaspoon of grocery-store extract!

MANUFACTURERS OF SAFE OATS

Gifts of Nature, Inc.

www.giftsofnature.net
810 7th Street E, #17
Polson, MT 59860
888-275-0003

Cream Hill Estates

www.creamhillestates.com
9633 rue Clément
LaSalle, Québec
Canada H8R 4B4
514-363-2066
866-727-3628

Gluten Free Oats

www.glutenfreeoats.com
578 Lane 9
Powell, WY 82435
307-754-2058

MY FAVORITE GLUTEN-FREE LIVING BOOK

Celiac Disease, A Hidden Epidemic *by Dr. Peter Green. Dr. Green takes the reader through the sometimes complicated and intimidating world of gluten-free living. The serious medical content of this book is softened by Dr. Green's straightforward, down-to-earth writing style. The questions and struggles of real patients peppered throughout the work put a human face on celiac disease.*

MY FAVORITE GLUTEN-FREE MAGAZINE

Living Without
www.livingwithout.com
PO Box 2126
Northbrook, IL 60065

ADDITIONAL RESOURCES FOR THE GLUTEN-FREE COMMUNITY

In addition to the national and local support groups, **www.celiac.com** *is a wonderful resource for medical studies, recipes, diagnosis steps, and more.*

My favorite on-line discussion board is http://forums.delphiforums.com/ celiac. *Very importantly, they have* adopted a "zero-tolerance" policy for inclusion of any gluten in the diet (i.e., picking croutons off a salad is not safe!). It is a great place to talk with other individuals who live the gluten-free diet every day. There is no fee for basic membership. Join in! Sometimes you will find me there!

Another very good on-line discussion board is www.glutenfreeforum.com.

For vacation getaways without worry, consider Bob and Ruth's Gluten-free Dining & Travel Club site, www.bobandruths.com. Members receive a quarterly newsletter that provides a variety of information to those on a gluten-free diet.

Note: Thousands of helpful organizations, companies, and web sites are available to the gluten-free community. Mountains of information are readily available. After getting safe at home, the next step should be joining a support group—whether national, local, or on-line—and learning more. And, if you're not the support-group type, start learning more by visiting the web sites included in this Appendix.

Index